Understanding and Supporting Bereaved Children

Andy McNiel, MA, is a co-owner of Satori Management and Consulting, LLC, providing education and consultation to the death, end-of-life, and bereavement fields. Andy serves the childhood bereavement field as a national fund-raiser, thought leader, and ambassador for issues related to childhood bereavement support, traveling extensively throughout the United States. Andy has served as a nonprofit manager and leader throughout his career, and has provided support and counseling to bereaved children, teenagers, and adults in a variety of support settings. He has served as chief executive officer of the National Alliance for Grieving Children, executive director of The Amelia Center in Birmingham, Alabama, and director of grief support services for Treasure Coast Hospice in Stuart, Florida. He is a national trainer for Boys and Girls Clubs of America and a member of the facilitator training corps of the American Foundation for Suicide Prevention. He is a nationally recognized presenter and trainer, using a balance of humor, teaching, and facilitating on a variety of topics related to strategic planning, nonprofit leadership, childhood bereavement support, adult bereavement issues, and group facilitation. He holds a BA in religion from Palm Beach Atlantic University and an MA in counseling from The University of Alabama at Birmingham.

Pamela Gabbay, EdD, FT, is a co-owner of Satori Management and Consulting, LLC, providing education and consultation to the death, end-of-life, and bereavement fields. Dr. Gabbay is an adjunct faculty member at Brandman University in California and is a member of the training corps for the American Foundation for Suicide Prevention. Formerly, Dr. Gabbay was the director of the Mourning Star Center for Grieving Children. She created and served as camp director for Camp Erin, Palm Springs, a bereavement camp for children. She served two terms on the board of directors of the National Alliance for Grieving Children (NAGC). Dr. Gabbay served as the president of the Southern California Chapter of the Association for Death Education and Counseling. Each year, Dr. Gabbay presents at multiple national conferences. She has presented at the annual conferences for the NAGC, the Association for Death Education and Counseling, the MISS Foundation, the American Association of Suicidology, Soaring Spirits Loss Foundation, and the Childhood Grief and Traumatic Loss Conference. Dr. Gabbay holds a Fellow in Thanatology certification from the Association for Death Education and Counseling and earned a master of arts degree in cognitive psychology from Claremont Graduate University. She earned a doctor of education degree in organizational leadership from Brandman University.

Understanding and Supporting Bereaved Children

A Practical Guide for Professionals

Andy McNiel, MA, and

Pamela Gabbay, EdD, FT

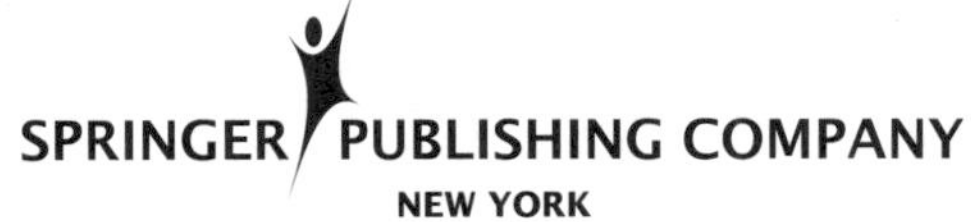

SPRINGER PUBLISHING COMPANY

NEW YORK

Springer Publishing Company, LLC
11 West 42nd Street
New York, NY 10036
www.springerpub.com

Acquisitions Editor: Sheri W. Sussman
Compositor: diacriTech

ISBN: 9780826140487
e-book ISBN: 9780826140494

17 18 19 20 21 / 5 4 3 2 1

The author and the publisher of this Work have made every effort to use sources believed to be reliable to provide information that is accurate and compatible with the standards generally accepted at the time of publication. The author and publisher shall not be liable for any special, consequential, or exemplary damages resulting, in whole or in part, from the readers' use of, or reliance on, the information contained in this book. The publisher has no responsibility for the persistence or accuracy of URLs for external or third-party Internet websites referred to in this publication and does not guarantee that any content on such websites is, or will remain, accurate or appropriate.

Library of Congress Cataloging-in-Publication Data
Names: McNiel, Andy, author. | Gabbay, Pamela, author.
Title: Understanding and supporting bereaved children : a practical guide for professionals / Andy McNiel and Pamela Gabbay.
Description: New York, NY : Springer Publishing Company, LLC, [2018] | Includes bibliographical references and index.
Identifiers: LCCN 2017013588| ISBN 9780826140487 | ISBN 9780826140494 (e-book)
Subjects: MESH: Grief | Child | Counseling—methods | Bereavement | Social Support | Attitude to Death | Child
Classification: LCC BF723.G75 | NLM WS 105.5.E5 | DDC 155.4/124—dc23 LC record available at https://lccn.loc.gov/2017013588

Contact us to receive discount rates on bulk purchases.
We can also customize our books to meet your needs.
For more information please contact: sales@springerpub.com

Printed in the United States of America by McNaughton & Gunn.

To my mother, Patricia Louise McNiel.
You were always my greatest encourager.
The memory of you continues to give me strength.
I miss you every day. To my dad, Winston McNiel.
You are a blessing to your family. Thank you for being you.
To my family, Dana, Bailea, Allyssa, and Naish.
You are my companions, my strength, and my hope.

—A. M.

To my parents, Jerry and Shirley Henry.
My greatest lessons came from the lives you lived and also from your premature deaths, which led me to this field.
To my husband, Richard, and my two children, Megan and Josh, and our extended family.
I couldn't imagine this journey without all of you!
I treasure your love and support.

—P. G.

Contents

Foreword

Many of us in the helping professions had solid academic or clinical training in our specific discipline or degree program—as social workers, counselors, chaplains, psychologists, school counselors, psychiatrists, clergy, or other mental health professionals. Yet, the majority of social service-oriented graduate degree programs, including the MSW, MA, PhD, EdD, and PsyD, as well as psychiatry, do not offer, let alone *require*, students to take at least one course related to grief and loss.

It is loss and grief—not always resulting from death, but also divorce, disappointment, abandonment, trauma, and other life experiences—that drive people to seek therapy, counseling, or therapeutic professional help in the first place, and often into the offices of those of us who care, but are untrained and unprepared.

The subpopulation of children and teens are often referred to as "the forgotten grievers." Yet we know that adverse childhood experiences, especially when unaddressed or unacknowledged, carry with them enduring negative consequences. We need to make understanding and responding to the needs of grieving children and teens a priority in our practices.

Whatever your professional setting, you will find the information in *Understanding and Supporting Bereaved Children: A Practical Guide for Professionals* accessible and applicable to your practice. Whether you consider yourself a grief counselor or a grief therapist, you are bound to encounter youth who are dealing with the aftermath of the death of a parent, sibling, or friend. This book will help you do so with more understanding, a solid theoretical foundation, and the skills needed to serve this vulnerable population. Andy McNiel and Pamela Gabbay know what they are talking about. With a combined 46 years of experience leading grief support programs, as well as teaching and training nationally in issues related to the needs of grieving children, they have been in the trenches: developing and running camps for grieving youth, guiding local and national organizations as thought leaders in the field, and counseling and providing support groups. Their collective insight, and the wisdom they have gained from listening to and interacting with grieving families, is a gift to all of us who want to improve our services.

In my 30-plus years with the Dougy Center—the first 5 years as a volunteer facilitator with our founder, Beverly Chappell, the next 25 years as executive director, and now in my final role as senior director of advocacy and training—I have trained, consulted for, and spoken to several hundred groups of professionals about the needs of grieving children. From teaching classes to psychiatry residents at Oregon Health Sciences University, to training the FBI's Rapid Deployment Team and the National Transportation Safety Board's Family Assistance staff, I found people hungry to do a better job providing quality services to children and their families after deaths that were both global and personal in scope. I wish I could have handed them this book!

Among the themes Andy McNiel and Pamela Gabbay weave throughout is the healing power of feeling understood, knowing you are not alone, and finding healthy forms of expression. They provide practical suggestions for ways in which you can incorporate these themes in your practice. Creating and making sense of our personal narratives and life stories is a life-long journey of discovery.

Over the past three decades, I have found myself in rooms in churches and homes and community centers and bereavement-support centers around the world, privileged to be trusted with some of the most raw and sacred expressions of grief known to humankind: socially stigmatized suicide-bereaved parents in South Korea; grief-stricken wives in Rikuzentakata, Japan, whose husbands were swept to sea by the March 2011 earthquake and tsunami; children whose parents died from cancer, car crashes, and diseases with names they could not yet pronounce; ten parents whose 6-year-olds were gunned down in their Connecticut classroom. More than 40,000 children, teens, young adults, and their parents or adult caregivers have shared their experiences after the death of a sibling, parent, or close friend in the years since the Dougy Center's founding in 1982. Primary and pressing among the topics of discussion in all of these groups, regardless of the cause of death or the culture, is this theme: *People don't get it*. The sentiment finds expression in words like, "Everyone's telling me to get over it." "It's hard to be around people because they want me to be happy." "Other people's lives are going on business-as-usual and mine has changed forever." We need to do a better job of *getting it*! The suggestions in this book will help us do so. This book fills a needed gap in the field.

Admittedly, the systems in which some of us work often foster a fix-it mentality, with managed care managers telling us how many sessions we may have with a client based on the American Psychiatric Association's *Diagnostic and Statistical Manual of Mental Disorders* (5th ed.; *DSM*-5; 2013) code we select as the label for symptoms we're seeing. Too often children are labeled (and overtreated pharmaceutically) as if their problems and behaviors are entirely inside their heads, as if they have "mental disorders." We see many children and teens with problematic behaviors directly resulting from the lack of social support, cultural understanding, and pressure to "move on." So if you are constrained by using *DSM* diagnostic codes in order to receive insurance reimbursement, please keep in mind that grief is not a disease or an illness to be cured. Grief is not a mental disorder, even though it is complicated, and those complications may compound healthy and adaptive outcomes. Those complications may be preexisting or new, including depression, anxiety, or escape-seeking behaviors. Other complications, equally impactful, may be the lack of support the child is receiving at school, in the home, from friends, or from the larger community.

I am not suggesting, nor are Andy McNiel and Pamela Gabbay, that the skills of being fully present, listening, and empathizing are always enough to help and support grieving children and teens. But these foundational skills are the building blocks to healthy grieving, along with helping children and teens to find their own forms of expression for coping with the death of someone in their lives and all the other changes that follow. I believe we often fail to provide healthy avenues for grieving, which result in behaviors frequently referred to pejoratively as *acting out*. Kids "act out" when their inner lives are not being listened to. The authors' passion to help professionals understand, rather than pathologize, is insightful, inspiring, and incisive.

The longer I do this work in this discipline of thanatology (the study of death), the more convinced I become that healing happens when we find others who will help us understand, make sense of, and find ways to express our experiences. This book provides a cauldron of ideas on how to assist children during some of the most difficult times in their lives. You can become one of the beacons of hope they remember as they process, and reprocess, the impact of these deaths on their lives.

Donna Schuurman, EdD, FT
Senior Director of Advocacy & Training
Executive Director Emeritus
The Dougy Center for Grieving Children & Families
Portland, Oregon

REFERENCE

American Psychiatric Association. (2013). *Diagnostic and statistical manual of mental disorders* (5th ed.). Arlington, VA: American Psychiatric Publishing.

Preface

Death is a natural part of life. It is one of the ultimate realities that bring us all together as human beings. Yet bereaved children often feel like they are the only ones dealing with the death of someone in their lives. This contribution to the field of childhood bereavement support is written as a practical guide for professionals to better understand how grief impacts the lives of bereaved children and how they can provide a safe place for grieving children and their families to find support. The information provided comes from our personal experiences working with children and their families over the past three decades.

Our lives and careers have been dedicated to supporting children, teenagers, and adults grieving the death of people in their lives. We believe that an informed, caring society is a better society and that we, as helping professionals, should be on the forefront of realizing this vision. We believe that all children should have access to supportive, compassionate adults in their communities. This book is written with the hundreds of children and families in mind whom we have had the sacred honor of walking alongside throughout our careers. We are dedicated to providing helpful information to professionals so children, no matter where they live, can find the support and understanding they need after the death of someone in their lives.

This book provides a theoretical model for understanding childhood grief resulting from death as a natural, transitional experience that is an integral part of a child's development into healthy adulthood. The experience of grief is personal to each individual, but, at the same time, is influenced by a variety of social, cultural, and environmental constructs. Professionals have a unique opportunity to walk with bereaved children and their families during some of the darkest times in their lives. When children are unsure about which way to turn, we can be there to encourage them as they find their way. When parents are unsure about how to help their children, or even how to help themselves, we can offer a safe place to pick up the pieces and learn to live even in the midst of grief and loss.

The ideas and examples provided in this book are taken from our years of experience providing support and counseling to bereaved children and their families in a variety of settings. Our experience has taught us that grief is not an illness in need of special treatment, but that it is an experience that bereaved children and adults must live. Over the past 50 years, a field of professionals and volunteers has emerged that is providing supportive care and counseling for bereaved children and adults. This care is not characterized by one singular human service field, but is a cross-section of many fields of care, including pastoral care, mental health, education, social work, health care, counseling, child life, and funeral service, to name a few. This book provides a construct that can apply in any of these settings as a compassionate approach to understanding and supporting bereaved children and their families.

The first five chapters provide a framework for understanding how grief impacts the lives of children and how their surrounding circumstances further influence their reactions to grief. The last five chapters offer a structure for professionals to provide support to bereaved children and their families. We detail factors that promote health in bereaved children, provide suggestions for creating a safe space for support, and outline modes of supporting bereaved children. Chapter 9 offers sample activities for each mode of support. Throughout the book you will find "How to Help" sections that offer practical ways professionals can be supportive to bereaved children and their families. It is our hope that this book will be a resource to professionals in their work with bereaved children and families and serve as a practical guide in the service you provide.

Acknowledgments

We would like to thank our colleagues and close friends Donna L. Schuurman, Albert Lee Strickland, Lynne Ann DeSpelder, Stephanie Gunner, Melissa Lunardini, and Lynn Snyder for their support and encouragement during this project.

A special thank you to Sheri Sussman and Mindy Chen from Springer Publishing for their guidance throughout the development and writing of this book.

Thank you to our many colleagues from the National Alliance for Grieving Children, the American Foundation for Suicide Prevention, the Boys and Girls Clubs of America, the Association for Death Education and Counseling, the National Funeral Directors Association, the National Hospice and Palliative Care Organization, and the Hospice Foundation of America. We appreciate your comradery and friendship. We are honored to serve bereaved children and their families alongside each of you.

Thank you to the children and families who have welcomed us into your lives—it has been our sacred honor to be a small part of your journey.

Thank you to the children and teenagers who contributed artwork to this book and your willingness to share a part of your story with us and our readers.

Thank you to our wonderful families for their love and support during our work on this book. It has meant more than you know.

CHAPTER 1

Understanding Childhood Grief and the Bereavement Support Professional's Role

When we are no longer able to change a situation, we are challenged to change ourselves.

—*Viktor E. Frankl*, Man's Search for Meaning

DEVELOPMENTAL FRAMEWORK FOR UNDERSTANDING GRIEF

Grief is a natural response to loss and a personal experience best understood from the perspective of the bereaved person. Because of this, finding a common language that addresses the unique and individual grief experiences of children can sometimes be challenging. Yet developing a framework for talking about childhood grief is important for further understanding the impact of grief on the lives of children.

Sigmund Freud (1917/1957) framed grief as a process of detaching energy from the deceased person and reinvesting that energy into other relationships. Freud believed that children lacked the libidinal ability to achieve this until much older into adolescence. Bowlby (1960, 1969), a student of Anna Freud, researched the reactions of infants separated from their primary caregiver, arguing that children as young as infants grieve the absence of a primary caregiver.

The seminal work on childhood grief specific to death loss, however, began with the Harvard Child Bereavement Study conducted by Silverman and Worden (1992). This study followed 125 parentally bereaved children and a matching non bereaved control group for 2 years. The Harvard Child Bereavement Study informed subsequent books and writings by both Worden and Silverman on the subject of childhood grief. Worden (1996, 2009) developed the Four Tasks of Mourning (see Table 1.1) as a framework for understanding the process of grief, which provided an alternative to viewing grief as a set of stages. Klass, Silverman, and Nickman (1996) were instrumental in the development of the concept of "continuing bonds." Silverman (2000) further expanded on this concept in her book, *Never Too Young to Know: Death in Children's Lives*. We discuss the concept of continuing bonds further in Chapter 7.

The works of both Worden and Silverman mark a shift in thinking about grief as a process of detachment from the deceased to one of transition into a new normal. In this way, the grieving person adapts to the changes brought about by the reality of the death and continues a meaningful connection with the deceased person through thoughts, internal conversations, memories, and legacy-honoring activities. Their work continues to inform the childhood bereavement field today in terms of theory and practice. Building on the constructs that Silverman and Worden have provided, we use a developmental framework to look at grief as a natural process of adaptation in which children, in the context of their family, community, and culture, transition from life before to life after the death of a significant person.

The childhood development theories of Piaget and Erikson provide a context for understanding normal childhood development. Its concepts are widely used today to shape the environments where children live, learn, play, grow, and develop. In addition to other environments where their theories have been applied, developmental theory provides a useful backdrop to understand how

Table 1.1 Worden's Four Tasks of Mourning

Task	Brief Description
To accept the reality of the loss	Accepting reality that the person died and will not return
To process the pain of grief	To feel the feelings of grief
To adjust to a world without the deceased	Adjusting to how the death impacts everyday life; one's own sense of self; and one's beliefs, values, and assumptions about the world
To find an enduring connection with the deceased in the midst of embarking on a new life	Finding ways to stay connected with the person who has died, but also to embrace new experiences and continue living life

Source: Worden (2009).

children experience grief and adapt to the changes that death brings to their lives. Using a developmental framework to understand childhood grief provides a common language, context, and construct for our discussion. More specific, Piaget's ideas surrounding adaptation of mental constructs or schemas (Piaget & Cook, 1952) and Erik Erikson's concepts of developmental tasks (Erikson, 1950, 1963) offer a framework for more fully understanding how children experience grief and adapt to the changes that death brings to their understanding of the world.

Applying Piaget's ideas about adaptation to our understanding of grief allows a better appreciation of the complexities being experienced internally by a bereaved child. Piaget theorizes that individuals possess schemas, or mental constructs, for understanding and interacting with the world around them. As a person encounters new experiences, over time these mental constructs are adapted by the processes of assimilation and accommodation. Adaptation is an ongoing process in a person's life that lasts throughout the person's lifetime, from the moment of birth until the moment of death.

For example, if a mom places a rattle in the hand of an infant, that child will instinctively close its tiny hand around the rattle and pull it toward her mouth. This is a schema called *grab and bite*. Now, imagine that mom is placing her infant on the floor on a blanket and her bracelet falls from her arm, catching the attention of her child. It is natural for the infant to reach out to interact with this new object in a way that is familiar to the child. So, the child is likely to use the existing construct of grab and bite to interact with the bracelet. Piaget calls this *assimilation*, the process of using an existing schema to adapt a new object or experience into our understanding of how the world works. In other words, the child assimilates the bracelet into her understanding of the world using the schema, grab and bite. Though not the correct use of a bracelet, grab and bite works nicely for the infant and there is no need to further explore the object in a different way.

Let's further imagine that this same infant encounters a beach ball. She might first attempt to interact with it using the existing construct, grab and bite, only to quickly realize that this existing schema does not work in this case. The ball is too large for successfully employing grab and bite in adapting this object into her understanding of the world. In order to fully adapt to this new experience, the infant must interact and struggle with the beach ball. Through this struggle the infant learns how the object reacts to her touch and in time might learn that the ball can bounce and that by using both arms, she can also hold the ball. In doing this, the infant has created an entirely new schema for interacting with the beach ball, called *hold and bounce*. This is the process of accommodation, reconfiguring, or constructing an entirely new schema or mental image in order to adapt a new object or experience into your understanding of how the world works. In others words, an infant creates a mental construct that will accommodate for this new object or experience.

The concepts of adaptation, assimilation, and accommodation, when applied to childhood grief, provide a context for more fully understanding a child's process of adapting the death of a parent, sibling, family member, or close friend to their understanding of the world. Imagine, if you will, that the beach ball is the death of a person close to the child and her struggle with the beach ball is her struggle with adapting to the reality that someone in her life has died. It is also the struggle to more fully understand what the death means to her life and how to adapt to a world in which this person is no longer physically present. In this regard, grief can be understood as a process of adaptation as children struggle to assimilate and accommodate their understanding of how the world works, their place in this newly discovered world, and their ability to successfully navigate the changes brought about by the death.

Erikson's (1950, 1963) developmental theory is framed by the concept that each developmental stage is marked by a task or crisis that the child must successfully navigate. Some children adapt in ways that are healthy and helpful, but others might struggle and develop what Erikson calls *maladaptations*. These are ways of adapting to life that are neither helpful nor healthy for a child. His theory suggests that there is also an array of psychological, social, emotional, cultural, and environmental factors that contribute to a child's ability to successfully navigate each stage of development. These include a child's temperament and personality, the child's relationship with caregivers, friends, and siblings, intelligence quotient, culture, community life, and home environment, to name a few.

Borrowing some of the language and framework of Erikson's developmental theory, we can further understand a child's reaction after the death of someone in the child's life as a natural process of development in which the child struggles with the crisis or task of adapting his or her ideals (how he or she believed the world to work) with the new reality (how the world really works). This process is further complicated by the age and ability of the child to understand important factual concepts about life. For example, Speece and Brent (1984) identified three realities about death with which younger children struggle: (a) that death is irreversible; (b) that when a person dies, his or her bodily functions also cease; and (c) that a person who is dead cannot communicate with them. We discuss these in more detail later in the text.

As children struggle with the task of accepting the reality of the death, they might adapt in ways that are helpful or harmful. In other words, they successfully adapt in healthy ways, or develop maladaptations that further complicate their situation. We explore more about these concepts in Chapter 6 when we discuss promoting health in grieving children and ideas for helping them deal with some of the complexities and challenges of grief.

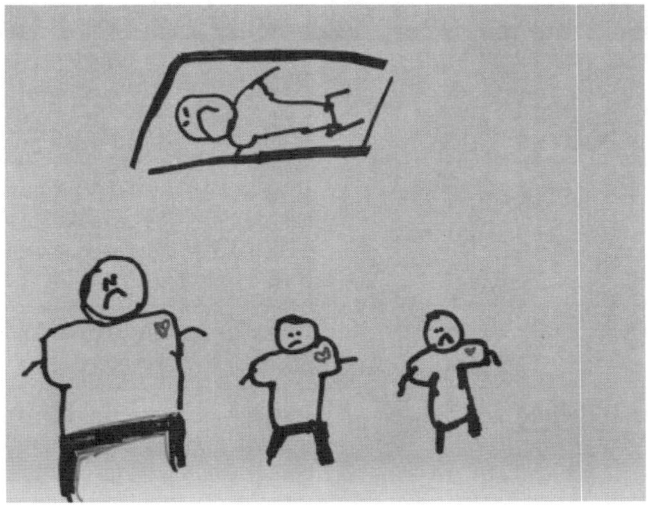

Figure 1.1 Artwork created by a younger child whose mom died.

We use both Piaget's and Erikson's concepts throughout this book to provide a framework and language for understanding how children experience grief, and how professionals can provide assistance as children grieve the death of a person in their lives (Figure 1.1).

FIVE UNIVERSAL REALITIES OF GRIEF

There are certain realities of grief (Table 1.2) that should also be considered in order to more fully develop a framework for understanding childhood grief and our role as professional helpers in the lives of children. Grief is an individual journey and we should be cautious about bringing too many assumptions into the counseling/support relationship with bereaved children and their families. We, the authors, operate from a theoretical framework for understanding childhood grief that encourages practitioners to recognize the individual nature of grief. In our extensive experience providing counseling and support to bereaved children, we have observed *Five Universal Realities* related to grief that we believe should be taken into consideration when providing a supportive environment to bereaved children. These realities have important implications on our relationship with grieving children under our care and apply equally to children, teenagers, and adults. In our estimation, these are the primary assumptions we should bring with us into the grief support and counseling relationship.

Table 1.2 Five Universal Realities of Grief

Universal Reality	Implications for the Professionals' Relationship With Bereaved Children
Grief is personal.	Therefore, the client is the expert of his or her own grief. The professional should avoid assumptions and approach the bereaved child as a learner.
Grief is transitional.	Therefore, children need the time and space to explore their new reality.
Grief is seen and unseen.	Therefore, professionals should avoid assuming whether or not someone is grieving based on outward expressions of grief.
Grief is a shared experience.	Therefore, professionals should find ways to incorporate and include parents in the support and counseling setting.
Grief is integral.	Therefore, it is not our role as professionals to take a child's grief away, but instead to provide a safe environment where children can struggle with their grief.

Universal Reality One: Grief Is Personal

Grief is personal; it belongs to the person who is grieving. Each person grieves and copes with grief in the way that feels most natural to that person. There is no right or wrong way to grieve. Children have their own unique personalities and preferences for how to interact with the world around them; this is also true when it comes to their grief. Children bring with them their understanding of the world, personality, cultural context, and beliefs. Understanding that grief is personal and belongs to the griever also has important implications on how we, professionals, interact with children who are grieving. It means we do not force help or support upon children, nor do we invade their space by assuming they want to talk to us about it. On the contrary, we enter that space as learners, and only journey with them as we are invited to do so. We expound on this and provide insight into how to create a safe supportive space for bereaved children in Chapter 7.

Universal Reality Two: Grief Is Transitional

Grief is transitional. This transition is both personal and corporate. It is personal as we see individuals adapt their own understanding of the world, how the world works, and their place in the world. It is corporate as we observe the transition of families as they restructure, regroup, and adapt to the absence of one of their primary members. People who are grieving are in transition from the way things were before the death of someone in their life to the way things are now that that person has died. Silverman (2000) defined grief as a non stagnant transition from one state of being to another.

This transition is a process that continues throughout children's lives. Since there is no specific timeline for grief, children will continue to grieve and regrieve, particularly as they reach important milestones in their lives like graduation, marriage, and having children of their own. Because of this, the purpose of grief support is not to find a remedy for grief. Instead, professionals should provide space for children to explore the changes that grief is bringing to their reality. We should offer information about the shared understanding of those grieving the death of someone in their lives, normalizing children's personal grief experiences. We best serve bereaved children when we reinforce coping skills and provide a space for expression, self-determination, and encouragement.

Universal Reality Three: Grief Is Both Seen and Unseen

The old adage, "the squeaky wheel gets the grease," is often true when it comes to grief. Children who outwardly display their grief often get the attention and concern of their caregivers, whereas children who are more reserved and less outwardly responsive might not get the same level of attention. It is easy to assume that children are okay if they are not showing a lot of outward signs of grief. At the same time, it is also common for adults to worry that children who are not outwardly expressing their grief are "bottling it up inside" or "holding it in." Yet, grief is not a simple surface experience that we express once, get out of, and then move on from. In reality, grief is an experience that often lacks a language and can, at times (particularly for children), be challenging to express. These internal experiences often are personal and not shared with others. It is important for us to remember that we do not know all there is to know about another person's grief. There are always those parts of grief that are that person's alone and may never find expression verbally or otherwise, but nonetheless are an important part of shaping who a person is becoming and how he or she will cope. Further, we should not assume that because a person is not outwardly expressing grief that he or she is "fine" and do not need support and understanding.

Grief is both seen and unseen. Recognizing this reality has implications on how we interact with children as professionals. For example, an internship student remarked during a clinical review meeting that she believed that a grieving child under her care no longer needed her help. This assumption stemmed from the fact that the child was not showing outward signs of grief in session and never talked about the person who died. Professionals should avoid the faulty assumption that, if a child is not talking about the person who died or the death, there is no need for counseling or support. Withdrawing support from a child risks leaving him or her to grieve alone and without the supportive adult presence needed by the child. It is important that professionals working with grieving children avoid such assumptions. Instead, we should focus on creating an environment that is comfortable to children and reflects compassion, care, and support.

Universal Reality Four: Grief Is a Shared Experience

Grief is a shared experience. Though grief is personal and belongs to the person who is grieving, it does not happen in a vacuum. Children receiving support or counseling are coming to this support from a particular culture, family, and community context. These factors not only influence children's understanding of the world, but also their understanding of death, and how they grieve and cope with its reality. As mentioned previously, the Harvard Child Bereavement Study identified the relationship with the surviving caregiver as a top indicator of the health of bereaved children after a death. Researchers at the Arizona State University Family Bereavement Program further substantiated the importance of the parent/child relationship as the single most important factor in a child's health after a death (Haine, Wolchik, Sandler, Millsap, & Ayers, 2006). Because of the influence that the parent–child relationship has on a child's well-being after a death, professionals should find ways to incorporate and include parents in the support and counseling setting. We further discuss ideas about how to do this in Chapter 8.

Universal Reality Five: Grief Is Integral

Grief is integral. By this, we mean that grief is an integral part of how a person incorporates the loss into his or her present reality. Another way to think about it is that grief is a process by which an individual struggles with a reality that does not have a context or, to borrow from Piaget, lacks a mental construct for understanding how to incorporate this new experience into his or her existing understanding of how the world works. As the individual struggles with the "beach ball" (the death of someone significant), the individual is learning how to adapt the experience of the death into his or her present reality and understanding of how the world works. This process is integral to a child's understanding of himself or herself, how the world works, and directly related to who the child is becoming and will be as a result of this event. So, our job as professionals is not to take a child's grief away, but to provide a safe environment in which the child can grieve (struggle with the beach ball). The struggle with grief is an integral part of a child's development of new mental constructs that enable adaptation to the reality of the death.

The terminology and language we often use to discuss grief in today's society describes grief in terms of symptoms, healing, and recovery and depicts grief as an illness to which we must seek a cure (Silverman, 2013). There is no shortage of attempts to label, name, articulate, and identify grief in all the ways it might manifest itself in a child's life. Our experience working with bereaved children and families over the years has taught us to use caution when trying to create a "one-size-fits-all" approach to understanding and helping bereaved children. Further, many of the constructs being used today to talk about grief imply that there are types of grief that require special treatment by experts. In no place is this better demonstrated than by the *Diagnostic and Statistical Manual of Mental Disorders* (5th ed.; *DSM-5*; American Psychiatric Association [APA], 2013) review committee's removal of the bereavement exclusion and the inclusion of Persistent Complex Bereavement Disorder in the "Areas for Further Study" section (APA, 2013). This move by leaders in the mental health community reflects a mischaracterization of grief as an illness for which we need to seek a cure. The problem is that there is not a cure for grief because grief is not something that needs to be cured. Grief is an integral, transitional human experience that children and families must live through as they adapt their loss into a new understanding of how the world works and of their place in that world (Silverman, 2013). It is the role of the grief support professional to be a sounding board, a caring presence to walk with bereaved children and their families, and to be a witness to their story and their pain.

The five universal realities of grief provide a context for understanding and supporting bereaved children and will be expounded upon throughout this text. Our contention is that caring for bereaved children begins with understanding that grief belongs to the griever and that grief is itself a healthy, integral part of helping children make the transition to a new understanding of how the world works; namely, that people in our lives can die and, at the same time, we can be okay and continue to live and thrive.

SPECIAL CONSIDERATIONS FOR TRAUMA

Trauma is a common human reaction to scary, violent, catastrophic, gruesome, inconceivable events. For example, Rick was in a car crash with his family. He was in the back seat sitting with his grandmother. She was badly injured from the accident and he held her as she died waiting for first responders. He reflected that, "Everything seemed to move in slow motion as I held my grandmother. There was a lot of blood and her eyes were open, but not looking at me. It seemed like it took forever for the ambulance to arrive. I can still see it in my mind like I am there. Sometimes I dream about it at night."

Cognitively, events that cause traumatic reactions in individuals are too much for our minds to quickly absorb, interpret, or adapt. These events are like an assault on our ideals and our assumptions about how the world works. It is important for professionals to note that whether something is traumatic or not is dependent upon the perception of the person experiencing the event. For example, one family member might watch a beloved person die and not be traumatized by it, whereas another family member witnesses the same death and experience symptoms of trauma.

Many people who manifest traumatic symptoms are able to adapt the experience in a healthy way (Bonanno, 2005). Others have a more difficult time and their trauma symptoms linger and intensify, requiring intervention and treatment. The various editions of the *DSM* have included a diagnosis for post-traumatic stress disorder (PTSD) with specific guidelines for diagnosis. The term *PTSD* has become common in news reports and magazine articles over the past 30 years and is sometimes used interchangeably with the term *trauma*. Professionals should use caution when referring to traumatic symptoms to not confuse common trauma reactions with a disorder diagnosis. Those suffering from PTSD require specific support and appropriate referral to treatment for this condition is vital. Although many individuals' trauma symptoms do not meet the criteria (duration and intensity) of a PTSD diagnosis, professionals should err on the side of caution and refer individuals with trauma symptoms to the appropriate professional for evaluation and assessment.

THE ROLE OF THE BEREAVEMENT SUPPORT PROFESSIONAL

Understanding our role as bereavement support professionals is paramount to providing bereaved children and their families with the care they need. The five universal realities of grief help us understand how we should approach the grieving person. Namely, we should approach grievers as learners and facilitators. After all, grief is not an illness that we are treating; it is a natural life experience that children and their families are living through. Throughout this book, we present information that will aid the bereavement support professional in helping children and their families impacted by the death of someone in their lives. Our role as professionals is threefold: (a) to directly support and care for grieving children; (b) to provide support to the parents, guardians, and caregivers of bereaved children; and (c) to provide information and resources to parents, guardians, and caregivers about how grief impacts their children and how *they* can help their children.

SUMMARY

Childhood grief is best understood as a natural response to loss. The professional should enter the support relationship with the assumption that children bring their own unique grief experiences with them. Grief is a transitional, personal, and integral experience that will ebb and flow in children's lives as they grow into adulthood. There are parts of a person's grief and story that they may never share with others. At the same time, grief is experienced within the context of families and is often steeped in culture and impacted by numerous internal and external factors. Grieving children sometimes experience trauma symptoms; appropriate referral and treatment for ongoing, persistent symptoms should be provided. Clearly understanding our role as bereavement support professionals is paramount to providing a safe space for bereaved children to express, work through, and cope with grief.

REFERENCES

American Psychiatric Association. (2013). *Diagnostic and statistical manual of mental disorders* (5th ed.). Arlington, VA: American Psychiatric Publishing.

Bonanno, G. A. (2005). Resilience in the face of potential trauma. *Current Directions in Science, 14*, 135–138.

Bowlby, J. (1960). Grief and mourning in infancy and early childhood. *Psychoanalytic Study of the Child, 15*, 9–52.

Bowlby, J. (1969). *Attachment and loss: Attachment* (Vol. 1). London, England: Hogarth Press.

Erikson, E. H. (1950). *Childhood and society.* New York, NY: Norton Publishing.

Erikson, E. H. (Ed.). (1963). *Youth: Change and challenge.* New York, NY: Basic Books.

Freud, S. (1957). *Mourning and melancholia.* New York, NY: Basic Books. (Original work published 1917)

Haine, R. A., Wolchik, S. A., Sandler, I. N., Millsap, R. E., & Ayers, T. S. (2006). Positive parenting as a protective resource for parentally bereaved children. *Death Studies, 30*, 1–28.

Klass, D., Silverman, S., & Nickman, S. (Eds.). (1996). *Continuing bonds: New understandings of grief.* Washington, DC: Taylor & Francis.

Piaget, J., & Cook, M. T. (1952). *The origins of intelligence in children.* New York, NY: International University Press.

Silverman, P. R. (2000). *Never too young to know: Death in children's lives.* New York, NY: Oxford University Press.

Silverman, P. R. (2013). Lessons I have learned. *British Journal of Social Work, 43*, 216–232.

Silverman, P. R., & Worden, J. W. (1992). Children's reactions in the early months after the death of a parent. *American Journal of Orthopsychiatry, 62*, 93–104.

Speece, M. W., & Brent, S. B. (1984). Children's understanding of death A review of three components of a death concept. *Child Development, 55*, 1671–1686.

Worden, J. W. (1996). *Children and grief: When a parent dies.* New York, NY: Guilford Press.

Worden, J. W. (2009). *Grief counseling and grief therapy.* New York, NY: Springer Publishing.

CHAPTER 2

Impact of Grief on Children

Grief doesn't have a plot. It isn't smooth. There is no beginning and middle and end.

—*Ann Hood,* Comfort

COMMON GRIEF REACTIONS IN CHILDREN

In our years of working with grieving families, we spent much of our time helping to educate family members and other caring adults about the experiences of children after the death of someone close. One misconception of many family members and adults is the notion that children grieve similarly to adults. Often, the perception of parents or caregivers is that children are "little adults" who are capable of managing their grief in quite the same way as an adult. Yet the bereavement of children is different than the bereavement of adults (Corr & Corr, 1996). Cognitively and intellectually they are still growing and developing and do not have the same amount of life experience as adults to adapt their grief in the same ways.

Another misconception on the opposite end of the spectrum is the assumption that children are not being affected at all, simply because they are too young to fully comprehend what is going on around them. However, children and teens have more awareness than most adults realize and they are affected by the death of someone close (Kastenbaum, 2000). Even if they do not fully understand what is happening around them, they are being impacted on many levels. The impact of the loss will be interpreted from the limited experiences and understanding of children and it will affect them for many years to come.

As you read these sections, keep in mind that grief is an individual experience and unique to each person's situation. These common reactions are generalizations that may or may not be applicable in every case. They are meant to provide a context for understanding how children react to the death of a person in their lives. As professionals caring for bereaved children, we should take the position as learners, allowing children to teach us about their unique grief experiences.

Emotional Reactions

Grief is frequently experienced and expressed through our emotions. Children often have a myriad of emotions after they hear the news about the death of someone close. These emotions can run the gamut from shock, numbness, confusion, disbelief, and sadness, to anger, rage, fear, and guilt. Closely following the death, some children are often silent or understated in their reactions and some might appear to not show any emotion at all. This does not mean that they are not affected or are not grieving; not showing emotion in the beginning can mean many things. It could be that children do not know how to express what they are feeling. They might be confused by what has happened and lack the words to express what they are actually feeling. Or they just might want their feelings to stay private. It is important to remember that private grief doesn't mean that there is no grief. It just means that children are choosing to keep it private at that point in time.

Children will also go in and out of emotions. There is no predictable pattern, no step by step guide. One minute, children might be laughing and playing and the next minute, appear sad and disconnected. For example, Jamie was 7 years old when his dad died of a heart attack. His teacher commented that he played with the other children just fine on the playground. But, after some time, she would notice that he was not with the other children. Scanning the yard, she would see him sitting on a swing, kicking the dirt with his shoes with a look of "deep thought" on his face. Similarly, children might be expressing their grief, but then suddenly switch gears and want to talk about something else completely different. All of these situations are common grief responses. It's difficult for children to sustain any one emotion for any length of time. This vacillation of emotional responses is common in children.

It is important to note that talking about their feelings is not the only way that children express their emotions. It is common for children to express their emotions in a variety of ways, not just by using words. For example, Lisa's mom died from cancer when she was 15. Before her mom died, Lisa was quite talkative. After her mom died, she became more quiet. Most days, she didn't feel like talking about her mom or her mom's death. Instead, she preferred to express herself through painting. When Lisa's mom was alive, she also liked to paint. In fact, Lisa and her mom spent a lot of time painting together, even after her mom got sick. Now Lisa likes to paint, both as a way of expressing herself and also as a way of feeling closer to her mom. Some other common ways children express their feelings of grief are through imaginative play, through sports or physical activity, through creativity (like painting, artwork), through music, or through writing, to name a few (Figure 2.1).

How to Help

Professionals can help children with emotional reactions to grief by providing space in the support setting for children to express their grief in healthy, safe ways. Three important ground rules to establish with children regarding expressing their emotions are as follows: (a) do not do things that hurt yourself (e.g., punching a wall, cutting), (b) do not do things that hurt others (hitting, calling names, etc.), and (c) do not destroy property (e.g., expressing anger by vandalizing property). Finally, professionals can offer support to children and their emotional expressions by providing suggestions of ways children can deal with intense feelings and stress. Sometimes children just need to have the space to brainstorm alternative ways to express themselves in ways that are safe.

Finally, professionals can normalize children's feelings by making space for the expression of any feeling a child might be experiencing, including anger, deep sadness, or guilt. Children are better able to handle their feelings when they experience understanding and patience from the adults in their lives. Professionals can ensure the support environment is free from judgement, as well as connect children with others who might be experiencing similar feelings.

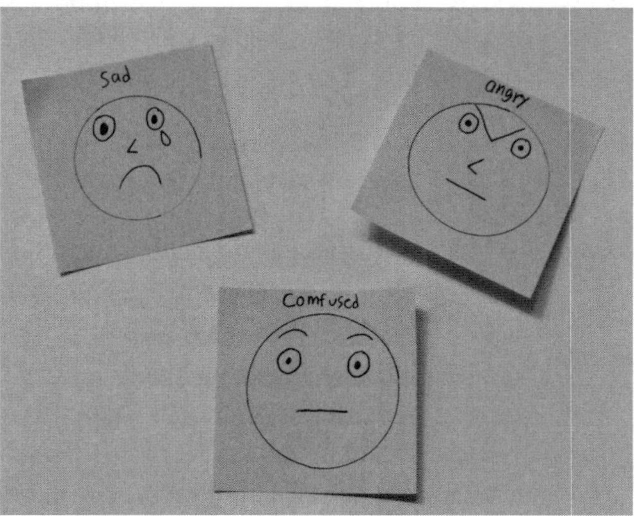

Figure 2.1 Artwork created by an older child whose dad died.

Physical Reactions

Grief is also physical. Like emotional reactions, physical reactions can vary greatly among children. It is common for children to have physical complaints of stomachaches, headaches, or nausea. Sometimes complaints will be strong enough that parents will take their children to the doctor. Over the years of providing support to bereaved children and families, we have had numerous families who were referred to us for support by their pediatricians for this very reason.

Another common physical reaction is for children to experience insomnia. Some children might feel like they are tired all of the time and cannot get enough sleep. Their appetite might also be affected, resulting in weight loss or weight gain. Some children are not hungry and lose their appetite, whereas others find that they have an increased appetite. Lethargy, or loss of energy, is also common. Just as with emotional reactions, these physical reactions can change from day to day or even hour to hour.

After a death, some children, particularly younger children, might regress. This could take the form of wetting the bed or wanting to sleep in the bed with their parent or caregiver. Younger children might return to thumb-sucking or speak using "baby talk." Regression occurs because children are striving to go

How to Help

Professionals can provide support to children in the area of physical reactions by providing activities and information in the support setting that offer suggestions about how to take care of oneself physically when one is grieving. Providing information to parents will help them to plan balanced meals at home and to better understand the physical reactions they might be seeing in their children. It can be helpful if parents take their children for a checkup with their pediatrician during this time. It is important that the pediatrician know all that is going on in their children's lives, so that the pediatrician can also monitor their physical health.

Regressive behaviors are rarely helped by punishment or trying to force a child back to more age appropriate behaviors. Regressive behaviors are best helped by families establishing routines, clear expectations, and compassionately holding everyone in the home accountable to these expectations. Professionals can provide information in the support setting for children and their parents to process the changes in the home and to establish new norms and predictability. In time, this will allow children to feel safe and most often they will return to more age appropriate responses.

back to a time before all of the changes happened when they felt safe. Or, like 5-year-old Haley, whose dad died in a car accident, children might become afraid of the dark and have trouble sleeping. Even though Haley had a night light in her room, she still wanted to sleep with her mom. For the first few months after her dad died, she would crawl into her mother's bed each night. Regressive reactions can be concerning to parents, but as the family develops new routines and rituals and restores existing routines and rituals, children often return to more age appropriate behaviors.

Mental Reactions

Grief has an impact on the cognitive functioning of children. After a death, children often have trouble concentrating or focusing (Silverman & Worden, 1992). This lack of concentration occurs at home and at school and this is one of the most common ways that grief impacts children. Children are often preoccupied with why school matters now that that someone has died. Thoughts such as, "My dad died. Why should algebra matter anymore?" When children are grieving, they have trouble thinking as clearly and staying as focused as they once did. This reaction is similar to how an Etch-A-Sketch® works (Do you remember these from your childhood?). When you shake the Etch-A-Sketch, everything drawn on the surface will disappear. This is how children's brains often feel when they are grieving, like someone has just taken their brain and shaken it; all of the information that was there previously is gone. Children report that this happens to them quite often during class or right before a test. All of the information that they thought was there no longer is.

Children also ruminate about what has happened. They think about and worry about who else might die. Children might also worry about dying themselves, thinking, "If my mom died, then I can die, too." Their sense of security may be shattered by what has happened, as well as their sense that the world is a safe and predictable place. Many of these common assumptions about life can be challenged. Sometimes, a sense of unfairness can permeate children's thoughts after a death. Children might wonder how life could be so cruel to them, directly impacting their sense of justice. For example, Mark was 13 years old when his dad died from a heart attack. The year after his dad died, Mark began high school. During his freshman year, Mark made the junior varsity baseball team. After he made the team, he felt the loss of his dad quite acutely. He felt an overwhelming sense of anger that his dad was not there to cheer him on and even wondered if his dad would be proud of him. Children will struggle with these types of mental constructs as they are adapting their understanding of the predictability and security of their world.

How to Help

Professionals can support children in their mental reactions by providing space in the support setting for children to express some of their ideas or thoughts about their life and about the person who died. As children have the opportunity to participate in activities in which they can remember the person who died, talk about the death openly without judgement, and express their thoughts, they are able to clear their heads of some of the distressing thoughts that might be consuming much of their energy. Also, as children are able to find outlets for their emotions and their physical reactions, they also might find that their cognitive struggles are lessened.

Professionals can also provide information to parents and teachers about children and the impact that grief has on their cognitive functioning. It is helpful for children if they can establish an understanding and plan with their teacher and school counselor for receiving support when they are struggling during class. Patience and understanding by the adults in a child's life are powerful tools in restoring a child's sense of equilibrium after the death of someone in their life.

Spiritual Reactions

Children will often have a spiritual reaction to loss. Bereaved children who have been raised with spiritual beliefs or raised going to church, synagogue, or mosque may begin to question those beliefs. Children may wonder, "Where is God now? How can God just take my dad from me? Doesn't God care about me and my pain?" Take, for example, 16-year-old Jordan, whose sister died in a car accident. Jordan had been raised going to church with his family and they were a family of strong faith. After his sister died, Jordan questioned everything, including where God was when his sister died. He wondered, "How could God let a 14-year-old die when she had the rest of her life to live?"

Sometimes these questions can cause children to question or turn away from their faith. Often, this crisis of faith ebbs and flows, changing and evolving over time, as children begin to resolve some of these questions and, ultimately, many return to their pre-death beliefs. For others, however, their faith beliefs are permanently altered by the death. Still others fall somewhere in between. Even children that have not been raised in a structured religious setting will have feelings about God and the afterlife after someone close to them has died.

> **How to Help**
>
> Professionals should follow clear boundaries when discussing spiritual reactions with children who are grieving. It is tempting to chime in with our own personal religious or spiritual beliefs, but just as it is inappropriate for us to tell children and their families how they should grieve, it is also inappropriate for us to proselytize a person when they are hurting and vulnerable. Also, long-held family beliefs can offer children an anchor during the turbulent times of their grief. It can be dangerous to try to replace these beliefs with those of your own, leaving them even more vulnerable and confused. Just because children are struggling with their beliefs does not mean that those beliefs are not ultimately helpful to them. Remember, part of the process of adapting is struggling—and it is often in this struggle that children establish their new normal. Professionals should refer families back to their faith communities to more fully explore their questions with faith leaders. In the support setting, however, professionals can create space where children can express, explore, and process their spiritual reactions free from judgment.

Some children and families turn to their faith even more after a death, especially if their church community was part of their primary support prior to the death. This faith community could very well be one of the main things bolstering them. In fact, some bereaved children report that their spiritualty helped them to cope in the wake of the death (Andrews & Marotta, 2005). A reminder, however, is that each child in a family might react differently in terms of their faith. Again, one size does not fit all. Keep in mind that each child within the same family can have different reactions from one another.

FACTORS THAT INFLUENCE CHILDHOOD GRIEF

A child's reactions to the death of someone close to him or her is influenced by a number of factors. Children's grief should be viewed through the lens of their environment, cultural and social context, and surrounding circumstances in which they live their lives on a daily basis. In addition, there are internal factors, like personality and the way they prefer to be in the world, that impact how they grieve. Understanding these factors will help professionals better understand the children they are caring for and supporting. The following are a few examples of factors that can impact how children react to and experience their grief.

Preexisting Relationship With the Deceased

An important factor that can influence a child's grief is his or her preexisting relationship with the deceased person. The Harvard Child Bereavement Study (Silverman & Worden, 1992) found a correlation between the preexisting relationship of the child with the deceased parent and the healthy expression of grief after the parent's death. The study found that children who had a positive experience with the deceased person prior to their death were more likely to remember the deceased person in a positive way. Further, these children fared better as they were able to more openly talk about the person who died and were able to open up to others in their family about their feelings.

Worden (1996) noted that children who had a warm, loving relationship with the person who died fared better in the long run than children who had a contentious relationship with the person who died. He observed that children who had a conflicted relationship with the deceased prior to his or her death tended to be more angry and reactive, moving toward more destructive behaviors (Worden, 1996). Some additional factors to consider about the preexisting relationship with the deceased person are: (a) the role this person played in the child's life, (b) how close the child felt to the deceased, and (c) whether the relationship was warm and loving or contentious and chaotic.

For example, Jason's dad was the primary person who tucked him into bed each night. They would read a story and sing songs. After Jason's dad died suddenly, Jason had a difficult time falling asleep because he missed the special time he had with his father. Similarly, children will grieve in different ways depending on how close they felt to the person who died. Children might experience a deep sense of sadness if they were close to the person who died because they miss that person's presence in their lives. At the same time, a child who was not close to the person who died might also experience a deep sense of sadness over the person's death and also over the loss of the opportunity to ever be closer to the person who died. In Chapter 8, we provide ideas and activities for helping children address *unfinished business* they might have with the person who died.

Culture

Cultural factors and cultural context both directly and indirectly impact the way children react to the death of someone in their lives. Culture encompasses a wide range of areas, including shared beliefs, customs, and arts to ways of living life, thinking, working, and building community. A child's culture has a strong influence on his or her perceptions of self, others, and his or her place in the world.

Every culture has its own set of customs and beliefs about death, grief, and loss (Parkes, Laungani, & Young, 2015). Some cultures may dictate how the body is disposed, either by burial or cremation. Cultural considerations include funeral rituals, accepted periods of mourning, expression of grief, and beliefs about the afterlife (Bowlby, 1980). After someone dies, many families experience a time of confusion and chaos. Often, cultural customs surrounding death and dying have predictable and prescribed rituals that have been passed down from generation to generation. For some children, the rituals and customs of their culture can seem reassuring and familiar at a time when everything feels strange and unfamiliar.

Because children grieve within this particular cultural context, professionals should create an environment that is both culturally sensitive and culturally aware. Being culturally aware is the first step toward cultural sensitivity. Cultural awareness is acknowledging our own biases and existing stereotypes that might exist within us and positioning ourselves as learners. As professionals, we should allow our clients to teach us about their world view, beliefs, and customs and allow our practices to be shaped by the cultures of those under our care. This includes our support space, materials, and resources provided to children and their families. We discuss this further in Chapter 8.

Social Interactions and Relationships

Children grieve in a social context as well. A child's social circle is comprised of their school, their peers, and their friends. After a death, a child's social circle often changes. Children struggle to feel understood; they often think that others can't possibly know what they are going through. Often, grieving children feel different after the death and feel that they no longer fit in. They grapple with feelings of whether or not they belong (Packman, Horsley, Davies, & Kramer, 2006). Sometimes they feel judged by others because of the death of someone close.

Friends are often at a loss for words and don't know what to say. Rather than be uncomfortable, sometimes these friends avoid the bereaved youth altogether. Other times, they simply drift away. For example, after Michelle's mom died, she had trouble connecting with her friends, even friends whom she had been close to since kindergarten. She felt that they could not understand what she was going through or what she was feeling. When she was around her friends, she felt like she was speaking a foreign language that no one else could understand.

Some bereaved children do receive the support of friends and that support is often beneficial (Schoenfelder, Sandler, Wolchik, & MacKinnon, 2011). Even when children have friends who stand by them, they still have difficulties.

Children who have had a parent die cannot understand or tolerate when their friends are getting mad at their own parents, especially if it's over petty things. They don't understand why their friends do not appreciate what they have. Another common situation that happens is that a bereaved youth's friends are often ready to move on to other topics much more quickly than the grieving child is. This can also cause disruption in the social circle, again reinforcing to the grieving child or teen that he or she is not understood.

Personality and Preferences

Children have their own personalities and their own preferences about how they are most comfortable being in the world. Some children might process their grief openly with others, whereas other children might prefer to process their grief internally (McNiel & Schuurman, 2016). Also, children might feel comfortable expressing their grief in different ways. Some children might move toward high energy types of activities to cope with their grief, whereas others find expression in arts, crafts, or other creative outlets. There is no one way children "should" process, express, or cope with their grief. It is important to keep in mind that a child's preferences can change from day to day. We should avoid the assumption that children who are more introverted and quiet will only find expression in quiet reflective activities, or that children who are more extroverted and talkative will only enjoy more expressive, high energy activities. Professionals should provide a variety of options to children in the counseling or support setting so that children can participate in the ways that feel most natural to them at the time.

Relationship With The Parent or Caregiver

One of the top predictors of a child's health after the death of someone in his or her life is the relationship the child has with the parent or caregiver. When children feel a connection to their parent or caregiver and they perceive the relationship to be positive, they are more comfortable expressing their grief openly and asking questions they might have about the death. Also, children with a positive relationship with their parent or caregiver often have their grief validated and feel less alone in their grief. We discuss this important relationship further throughout the book and suggest ideas about how professionals can help to foster a positive relationship between parents and their children.

Past Experiences of Loss

There is a saying that goes, "When we don't know what to do, we do what we know." This is very true when it comes to a child and grief. If we put this in the context of Piaget's ideas about adaptation, this is a prime example of the difference between assimilating (adapting a new object or experience by using an existing construct) and accommodating (struggling with and creating an entirely new construct in order to adapt a new object or experience). A child's past experience with loss provides the context in which he or she might cope with, react to, or express grief. That is not to say that a child does not struggle with grief if the child has had multiple past losses because each loss has its own unique set of circumstances. Children who have had multiple losses, though, have a context for understanding the death of someone in their lives. In the same way, a person who is experiencing his or her first significant loss will not necessarily struggle more than someone who has had multiple losses, but that person does lack a context for the experience of grieving the death of someone in his or her life. In addition, a child might pull from other loss experiences that are nonbereavement, or from the example of a surviving caregiver who is coping in healthy ways.

Secondary Losses

The death of someone can result in secondary losses for children. Secondary losses develop as a result of the primary loss (Rando, 1993). Families sometimes have to move after a death, resulting in children having to change schools, make new friends, and leave behind their familiar surroundings. If the person who died was the primary source of income, families might lose financial stability, impacting children's sense of security and the loss of particular comforts once afforded them. These types of secondary losses become additional circumstances to which children must struggle to adapt. They become interwoven into their grief and impact children's reactions to the death (Mahon, 1999). Artwork, writing, and sharing in support settings will often reflect these types of challenges.

Gender

Gender also has an impact on how children grieve the death of someone in their lives. Society establishes cultural norms around gender that impact how children grieve the death of someone in their lives. When raising children, parents often socialize children differently when it comes to learning about death and grief (Silverman & Worden, 1992). Society will often assign both feminine and masculine ways of grieving, which can directly impact the way a child expresses and copes with grief. For example, cultural ideas that boys don't cry or that girls are more emotional than boys can place an unnecessary burden on a child to react in a particular way after a death. In an attempt to be strong, boys might internalize their feelings of sadness, instead expressing it as anger, which is a more socially accepted reaction in boys than that of sadness. Professionals should be careful, however, not to assume particular types of reactions are based on a person's gender.

Family Dynamics

Families are the context in which children develop their self-image, sense of humor, personal preferences, and a sense of their place in the world. Whatever the setting, when a family member dies, each individual in the family is struggling with how this loss impacts his or her self (Walsh & McGoldrick, 2004). In addition, the family unit as a whole struggles to adapt to the loss corporately. Most families function within the context of various domains that include roles and responsibilities, rituals and routines, expectations and values, beliefs and superstitions, and environment and interactions. Professionals working with bereaved children and their families should consider these five domains in their planning, preparation, and delivery of support services.

The Five Domains of Family Dynamics

Roles and Responsibilities

Each member of the family makes up an integral piece and part of the family whole. Families develop in such a way that individual members take on different roles and responsibilities that impact the family collectively. A family member's death creates a void in the roles and responsibilities held by that particular member of the family. For example, if a father whose primary role was to entertain the children, and whose primary responsibility was to manage the finances dies, the family will struggle to reshape itself to absorb the loss of those roles and responsibilities.

Similarly, surviving family members might struggle with their own place within the family as everyone shifts in reaction to the absence of this important person in the family unit. As these shifts are occurring, remaining family members typically take on additional roles and responsibilities in order to fill the void of the missing family member. Some grieving children will strive to take the place of the missing family member (Silverman, Baker, Cait, & Boerner, 2002–2003). Children might be doing this consciously or unconsciously. At the same time, they are grieving the death of a significant person in their lives. Grief takes a large amount of energy and this can be exhausting both cognitively and emotionally to everyone in the family. These factors create an added challenge for individuals as they experience these changes and the new reality that death has brought to their family. Research has shown that bereaved children will fare better based on the ability of their parent to adapt to these new roles (Silverman & Worden, 1992).

Rituals and Routines

Families also operate within a rhythm of rituals and routines. Routines are the daily activities that encompass the lives of families and bring a sense of predictability and stability to the family unit as a whole. *Rituals* are defined as regular weekly, monthly, or annual observances that are rich with meaning, and often steeped in history, tradition, culture, or strongly held beliefs. Rituals provide a context for celebrating, commemorating, worshipping, or honoring. When a family member dies, rituals are often enacted for the purpose of remembering, celebrating his or her life, and mourning his or her death. Other rituals become challenging as they might highlight the absence of the person who died. Some examples of these include that person's birthday, Thanksgiving, or other shared family holidays.

Routines are often impacted by the death of a family member. Sometimes they are completely derailed due to both the deceased's absence and the grief reactions of those remaining family members. For example, if the person who died regularly took the children to and from school, children might wonder and worry how they will get to school. Similarly, routines might be impacted because of the grief of individual family members and the lack of energy to maintain the pace of normal routines. For example, after the death of a spouse, the surviving parent might struggle with keeping up the normal routines, drained of energy from his or her own grief. It is important to remember that this is a common experience for bereaved people and that bereaved individuals need professionals to demonstrate compassion and understanding around these challenges.

At the same time, routines are important to the health of a child. As professionals, we should provide support and encouragement to parents and caregivers to maintain existing routines when possible and to develop new routines when old ones cannot be sustained. Children thrive in environments that are predictable where they know what to expect next. The death of someone in a child's life temporarily impacts their sense that the world is safe and predictable. Because of this, routines are an important part of restoring a sense of predictability and safety. We discuss this in further detail in Chapters 6 and 7 when we more closely examine the topics of promoting health in bereaved children and creating a safe space for support.

Expectations and Values

Just as children thrive in environments with strongly established routines (predictability and safety), children also thrive in environments with clearly defined expectations and values (what is expected of them and their behavior within the family). Children need adults to hold them accountable to operate within established expectations and to live out their shared family values. Maintaining existing expectations and establishing new expectations and values can be quite challenging for parents and caregivers, particularly when they too are grieving the death of someone in the family. A surviving spouse, or parents grieving the death of a child, might struggle with holding their children responsible for their behavior. As a result, it is common for bereaved children and families to struggle with issues of misbehavior, lack of discipline, and poor accountability.

Offering information and resources regarding setting boundaries, expectations, and discipline to parents and caregivers raising bereaved children is an important part of providing education and support to bereaved families. Children need the adults in their lives to hold them accountable for their behavior, even in the midst of their grief. Professionals can provide encouragement that bolsters the confidence of parents to both acknowledge their children's grief and at the same time provide the discipline needed for healthy growth and development.

Beliefs and Superstitions

Beliefs within the family are deeply held thoughts and ideas about how we live our lives, interact with others, behave responsibly, and frame religious or spiritual experiences. Beliefs are ways we define what is good, right, wrong, valuable, and important to us. Strongly held beliefs are often challenged by the death of someone in our life. For example, a child who has been taught within their family that God is good might question, "How can God be good if my sister has died?" In this the child might struggle to reconcile how God can be good and at the same time his sister can die.

Superstitions are beliefs that are frequently steeped in fear and that often associate certain behaviors with good or bad luck, or magical thinking. For example, one might believe that if he or she is a good person, then bad things won't happen to him or her. As a result, a child might think, "I must be bad because my dad died." The belief that they are somehow to blame for the person's death is a common reaction in children, particularly younger children. Children will not always verbalize this to the adults in their lives. Subsequently, they might struggle with guilt over the belief or superstition that they are somehow responsible for that person's death.

Professionals can model and encourage respectful communication and dialogue while families grapple both individually and as a group with reconciling deeply held beliefs in light of the reality of their loss. It is not the professional's role to challenge, replace, or establish family beliefs. On the contrary, professionals should respect the beliefs of their clients while providing a context for their clients to examine beliefs and superstitions that might be causing additional distress.

Environment and Atmosphere

Home environments are both the physical and emotional space within which the family interacts with one another. Home environments might vary from chaotic and high energy, to more reserved and mundane. The atmosphere or emotional space is generated by the general mood of the household, and the collective affect of the individuals within the family. The home environment and atmosphere can have elements of dysfunction or stability, or even both. The environment and atmosphere of the home can also contribute to the sense of safety felt by the children and other members of the family. Every member of the family contributes to the family environment and atmosphere, but the parents or caregivers tend to have the greatest influence on the atmosphere. Children will mimic the behaviors, affect, and mood posited by their caregivers (Figure 2.2).

When a family member dies, the emotional environment can become fractured or compromised because individuals within the family are grieving and because of the void that might be left by the deceased's absence. Feelings of shared sadness and loss might permeate the environment, bringing melancholy to the general mood of the family. Because parents have such a strong influence on the atmosphere of the home, the death of a parent particularly will impact both the physical and emotional environments. It is particularly

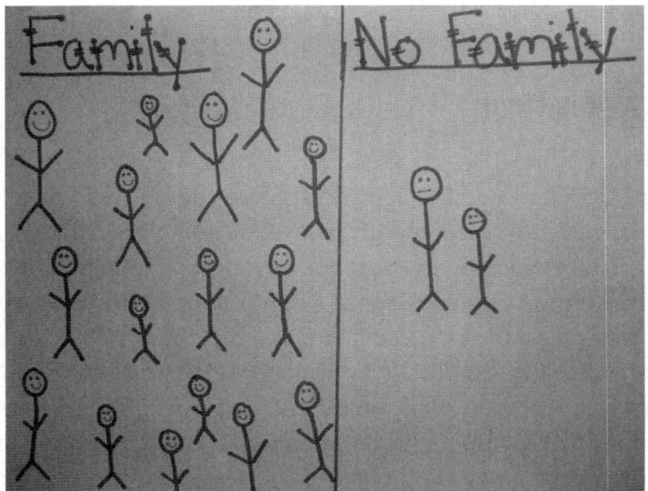

Figure 2.2 Artwork created by a child whose dad died.

challenging for a surviving spouse to maintain the preexisting physical and emotional environment in the absence of the deceased, and within the shifting moods and reactions to grief. Because children learn by example, they will be influenced and affected by how their parents and the adults around them are expressing their grief (Gilbert & Murray, 2007).

Professionals should consider the family's environment and atmosphere when providing support and counseling to bereaved children and their families. As mentioned previously with other aspects of family dynamics, it is not the place of the professional to pass judgment, or to attempt to manipulate the environment and atmosphere. We should, however, provide a supportive and therapeutic setting that acknowledges the importance of our physical and emotional environments. This allows children, parents, and families the opportunity to explore how the atmosphere of their home impacts their grief and how their grief has impacted the atmosphere of their home.

Our families are one of our primary sources of support throughout our lives. The death of a family member impacts every member of the family. After a death, a child's family changes, as do many of the preexisting family dynamics. One of the factors that will affect a child's grief is the child's family's patterns of living and ways of communication (DeSpelder & Strickland, 2015). Family dynamics are important because children model what they see in the adults around them. Not just their immediate family, but also in their extended family of aunts, uncles, and grandparents. As professionals providing care to children and their families after a death, we should consider the Five Domains of Family Dynamics in our planning and service delivery. We look more closely at how children are impacted by the death of a family member in Chapter 4 and explore ways to support healthy adaptation within the family unit (see "Parent/Child Adaptive Tasks").

Age and Maturity Level

The age and maturity level of a child directly impacts the child's grief. Children are at different developmental stages at different ages. Their developmental stage is also impacted by their maturity level as some children will move in and out of stages more rapidly than others. It is important to note for bereaved children that when they first experience a death they are in whatever stage of development they might find themselves, much like their friends around them. However, as a result of the death, children are often confronted with a reality much different than the one where they currently resided. They now know something about life that other children their age do not know in the same way they do. Because of this, they might be dealing with concepts and experiences beyond their current stage of mental development. In our experience working with bereaved children, we have seen children propelled into a higher level of mental development as a result of their situation following the death of someone in their lives.

It is also important to note that it is not our role as professionals to move children through developmental stages, or to get them to understand concepts that are beyond their ability to comprehend at the time. Children will naturally come to understand these concepts as they struggle with and interact with the world around them. It is our role, however, to provide encouragement, support, and tools for coping as children struggle to adapt to the new reality that the death has brought to their lives. Children are forever changed by a death and this cannot be separated from their natural developmental process. In other words, a child's grief becomes integrally intertwined with their developmental process.

Birth to 2 Years Old

Concept of Death

Babies do not have a cognitive understanding of death. They live in the present and understand their world according to who is around them at any given moment. They are affected by the moods and behaviors of others, especially when people in the household are upset. They are preverbal and have limited language skills to express what they are feeling.

Common Grief Responses

Even though babies and toddlers do not understand the concept of death, they do understand missing someone who was here before and no longer is. In response to a missing caregiver, they want to be held and comforted. They search and long for that person and may become irritable and unsettled because of the absence, leading to crying bouts. They can also become anxious and worried. This can lead to trouble with sleeping and loss of appetite.

For example, when Bailey's dad died he was only 1 year old. He cried a lot, missing his dad. He became clingy to his mom and wanted to be held all of the time. Each time he heard a man's voice, he turned his head to see who it was. Each time that he realized it was not his father, he began to cry.

3 to 5 Years Old

Concept of Death

Like babies, preschoolers have little or no concept of death. They also do not fully understand the permanence of death. They do, however, have language skills to express themselves and they know when someone is missing (Figure 2.3). Preschoolers view death as reversible and ever changing. This concept of death is reinforced by cartoon characters that children of this age often watch. A cartoon character falls from a cliff, seemingly to his death. In the very next scene the same character is alive and well. This type of scene illustrates the way children of this age conceptualize death.

Common Grief Responses

It is typical for grieving preschoolers to keep asking the same questions over and over again. Even though they have been told that, "Daddy has died and he is not coming home," they might still repeatedly ask, "When is Daddy coming home?" or "When is Daddy done being dead? I want him to come and play with me." These questions are commonplace and will continue until the child becomes mature enough to understand that daddy is not coming home. Children of this age will also repeat information that they have overheard, trying to make sense of it. Magical thinking often occurs during this time, as well. Magical thinking is the belief that they had some control over what happened to the deceased. For example, a young child might think that if he had been good and eaten all of his vegetables, his dad wouldn't have died.

Children of this age will also vary in their grief responses. Some will have intense periods of crying followed by periods of acting like nothing has happened. Others will regress in their behaviors such as bedwetting or not wanting to sleep alone. Also at this age, children will talk about the death like it is commonplace, even with strangers. For example, when Felicia was 4 years old her mom died from a brain aneurism. When Felicia's dad took her to the grocery store, Felicia asked every stranger that she encountered, "Did you know that my mommy just died?"

6 to 8 Years Old

Concept of Death

Younger school-aged children are in the early stages of understanding the concept of death, although for some in this age group, death is still seen as reversible and not permanent. They are beginning to think about what it means to be dead. This age group also imagines death as something that happens far away from them, for example, only to older people. If the death is someone close, they might think that they were responsible. They also have a personification view of death, visualizing death as a ghost or the bogeyman. This age group tends to be very literal and concrete in their thinking about death.

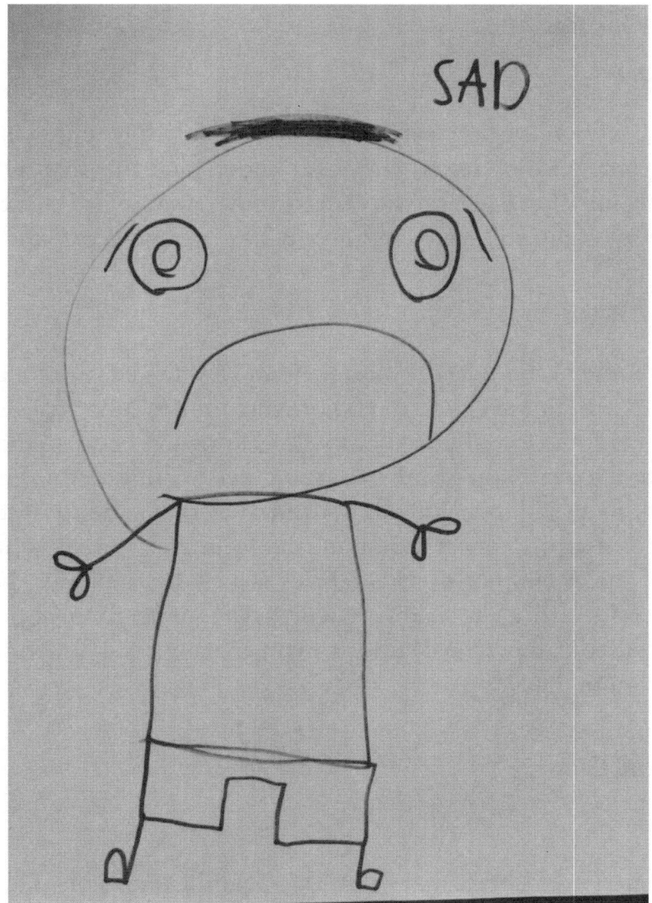

Figure 2.3 Artwork created by a younger child whose cousin died.

Common Grief Responses

Children in this age group are often concerned with the body and what happened to the body. They are worried that they might die, or someone else they love might die. Like younger kids, they have magical thinking about the death and the person that died. Because they often feel responsible for the death (even when they are not), they might make statements such as: "I was mad at my dad; I know that's why he died."

For example, Joseph had just learned to write when his brother died from leukemia. One day he asked his mom how to spell the word *dead*. Once she told him how to spell it, he proceeded to write it over and over again.

9 to 11 Years Old

Concept of Death

By the time children are between 9 and 11 years old, they understand the concept and permanence of death. They also understand that death is universal. Even though they have a more advanced understanding of death than their younger peers, many still have child-like beliefs around death and dying.

Common Grief Responses

Similar to younger school-aged children, 9- to 11-year-olds are concerned with the body and what happens to the body when it dies. It is typical in this age group to ask a lot of questions about what happened because they want the details about the death. Like younger school-aged children, this group is worried about who else in their life might die and also whether or not they could die. This age group is concerned about the feelings of others who have also experienced the death. For example, Erica is 10 years old. Her dad died last year from suicide. Erica has been very worried about her mom and the fact that her mom could die, too. One of Erica's main concerns is who would take care of her if her mom died?

12 to 14 Years Old

Concept of Death

This age group understands that death is final and irreversible. This age group also understands the universality of death and that it can happen to anyone. They are beginning to understand the abstract concept of death. They also want to know the details about the death and what occurred; however, they don't ask as many questions about what happened to the body. It is common in this age group, similar to older teens, to wonder what happens to people after they die.

Common Grief Responses

Young teens often do not want anyone to know that someone in their life has died. They do not want to be seen as different or vulnerable. They do not want people staring at them and they do not want the questions that often accompany the death of someone close. They might act as if nothing happened. They might also wait until they are at home and away from friends to show any emotion. They might also use jokes and humor to hide feelings of sadness.

For example, Kyle was in eighth grade when his dad died from cancer. Although his teachers and school counselor knew that his dad had been sick, he didn't want his mom to tell the school that his dad had actually died. He didn't want to be known as "that kid whose dad died" (Figure 2.4).

15 to 18 Years Old

Concept of Death

Teenagers have a more adult, abstract concept of death. By this age, they understand that people die and it's not possible to predict who is going to die. Teenagers have developed a more personalized view of death and it is not only seen as something that happens to others. Conversely, however, the reality of death in their lives is a direct contradiction to a teen's worldview that the teen is invincible. Like younger teens, older teens question what happens to people after they die.

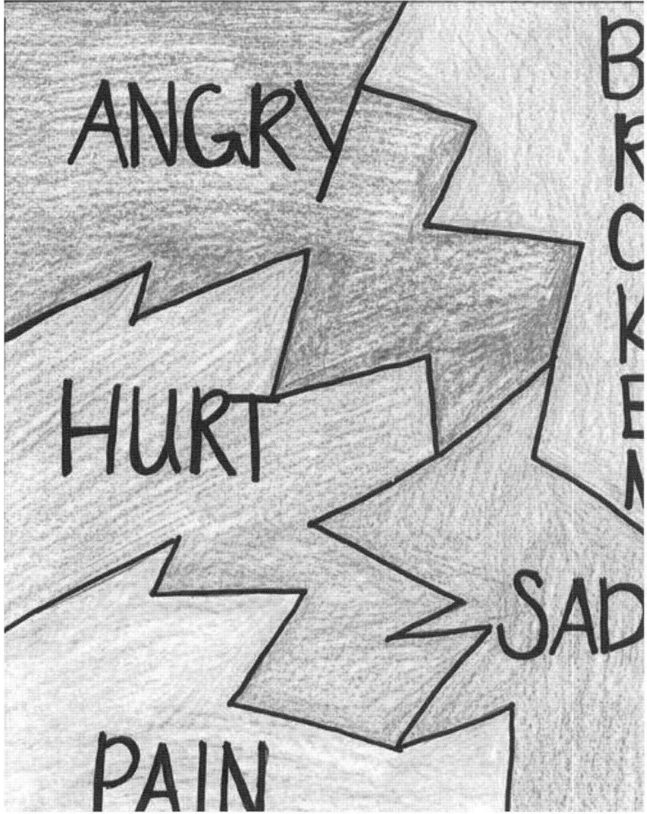

Figure 2.4 Artwork created by a teenager whose dad died.

Common Grief Responses

Reactions may vary with teens. Similar to adults, some teens may show a lot of emotions after a death, whereas others may not show many at all. Some older teens, like younger teens, will want to grieve privately because they don't want to be seen as different. They want to appear as though they have everything under control. This age group often pulls away from family and turns to their peers for support. Many will offer to take on adult responsibilities, believing that it is their duty to do so.

For example, after Monica's mom died, she turned to her friends for comfort. She didn't want to upset her dad because she knew that he was hurting a lot and missing her mom. She wanted to help her dad in some way. She began getting up early to make breakfast for her two younger siblings. She also made sure that they were dressed and ready for school before she left for high school (Table 2.1).

Important Consideration for Professionals

In our experience working with children and their families, we have observed that parents are often worried about their children's developmental well-being. Though they might not express it in those terms, parents are concerned that the death will have a negative impact on their children's ability to grow into healthy, functioning adults. Professionals have a unique opportunity to be an encouragement to parents by providing information about how grief impacts the lives of children. In addition, parents are encouraged when professionals reassure them that the death of someone in their children's lives does not have to so adversely affect them as to derail their future. Professionals can reassure and bolster the confidence of parents by providing insight into how parents can encourage, support, and connect with their children (see "Parent/Child Adaptive Tasks" in Chapter 4).

Table 2.1 Concept of Death and Grief Responses for Bereaved Children and Teenagers

Age	Concept of Death	Behaviors/Grief Responses
Birth–2 years old	No cognitive understanding of death Live in the present Affected by others around them Do not have the language skills to express themselves	Unsettled, irritable, crying Searching and longing Might become anxious and worried Want to be held Trouble sleeping or eating

(continued)

Table 2.1 Concept of Death and Grief Responses for Bereaved Children and Teenagers (*continued*)

Age	Concept of Death	Behaviors/Grief Responses
3–5 years old	Little or no cognitive understanding of death Do not understand the permanence of death Understand someone is missing Death is seen as reversible Think of death in terms of cartoon characters who can spring back to life at any time	Asks repeated questions such as "When is Daddy coming home?" Will repeat what others have said trying to make sense of it: "Did you know my mommy just died?" Magical thinking and acting Intense periods of crying followed by periods of acting like nothing happened Regression in behaviors
6–8 years old	Early stages of understanding the concept of death For some, death is still seen as reversible and not permanent Personification of death Feeling responsible for the death Think that death happens primarily to older people	Concerned with the body and what happened to the body Some will ask a lot of questions, whereas others will be more silent Magical thinking and acting Worried who else might die Worried that they may die Might make statements like, "I was mad at him, that's why he died."
9–11 years old	Understand the concept of death Understand the finality of death Understand that death is universal Still have many child-like beliefs around death and dying	Concerned with the body and what happened to the body Will ask a lot of questions seeking details about the death Concerned about the feelings of others Worried who else might die Worried that they may die
12–14 years old	Understand that death is final and universal Beginning to understand the abstract concept of death Want to know the details about the death Wonder what happens to people after they die	Might not want others to know that someone died Do not want to be seen as different Might act as though nothing happened and seem indifferent Might use jokes and humor to hide feelings of sadness
15–18 years old	More adult concept of death Ability to understand abstract concepts Have developed a more personalized view of death The reality of death contradicts a teen's worldview that the teen is invincible. Wonder what happens to people after they die	Reactions vary. Some are more likely to show shock, sadness, anger, whereas others will grieve privately Might pull away from family Often turn to peers for support Might want to take on more adult responsibilities Want to appear as though they have everything under control

WHAT BEREAVED CHILDREN WANT ADULTS TO KNOW

Their Grief Is Long Lasting

There are a number of misconceptions that adults often have regarding childhood grief. As professionals, we have an opportunity to provide parents and caregivers with information to clarify how grief impacts children. We can advocate for the children under our care by sharing accurate information with the adults in their lives that the children would want them to know.

Grief is not an experience that children have for a short period of time. They do not simply "get over" their grief, or "move on" from their grief after a few weeks or months. Grieving children do not forget the person who died as time passes. They might not think about the person or experience intense feelings of grief as often, but this does not mean they are not grieving the person who died. On the contrary, children will grieve the person who died for the rest of their lives. They will continue to think about the person and to experience grief over the person's death in different ways at different times as they experience each new stage of their lives.

As professionals, we can create understanding around this idea and help the adults in children's lives appreciate the enduring nature of grief in a person's life. We can normalize children's experiences by creating opportunities to acknowledge their ongoing relationship with the person who died and the bond that continues with that person even beyond their death. These continuing bonds might reflect a loving, caring relationship with the person who died, but can also manifest feelings of anger or hurt if the child's relationship with the person who died was contentious or strained. Either way, it is normal for children to transition their relationship with the person who died from one of physical presence to one of memories or sensing a person's presence with them.

They Cope With Their Grief Through Play

Children are not like "little adults." Children cope with grief differently than the adults in their lives. This sometimes creates misunderstanding among parents or caregivers that if children are playing and having "fun," then they are not grieving. This could not be further from the truth. Play is how children learn, grow, discover, express, and experience the world around them. This is no different after a person in their life dies. Children will use their play as a way of coping after a death. Play can also provide an outlet for expressing grief by exerting some of the high energy associated with some of the more intense feelings of grief children might be experiencing. Unlike adults, children are not capable of sustaining long periods of grief. Instead, they will come in and out of grief and in between they use play as a way to cope with their grief and to take a break from their grief.

As professionals, we should ensure that the support environment has opportunities for children to play. As we discuss in Chapter 8, there should be a variety of play options in which children might choose to participate. Play is also a great way for adults to connect with children and be invited into their world. We share ideas about how to engage with children in play in Chapters 7 and 8.

They Will Always Miss the Person Who Died

Somewhat related to the enduring nature of grief is the reality that grieving children continue to miss the person who died. In our work with grieving children over these many years, we have encountered families who were given poor advice by family, friends, and even professionals that they need to try to stop thinking about the person who died. On several occasions families have shared with me that their child's counselor suggested that they remove all pictures of the person who died and stop talking about them. This advice is not only in error, but can alienate children from the caring adults in their lives. Removing pictures and not talking about the person who died does not remove the thoughts of the person from a child's mind. It simply means they will stop talking to the caring adults in their lives about their grief or the person who died. This can leave a child to grieve alone without the support of the caring adults in their lives.

Sometimes They Want to Talk and Sometimes They Do Not

Support settings should provide opportunities for children to talk about their grief. Though there has been much improvement over the past 40 years with how we address death, dying, and bereavement with children in our society, there are still too many occasions when the needs of children are ignored and they are left out of family conversations on these topics. Too often, children hold their thoughts and feelings inside rather than sharing them with the caring adults in their lives. Professionals should invite children to share openly about their grief and we should educate parents about how to connect and communicate with their children on these very difficult topics.

Equally important, though, is to recognize that many children are not comfortable talking about their grief. Children also find expression of their grief through art, high energy activities, make believe, and other types of play. So our support settings should offer a variety of options for interaction with other children and with supportive, caring adults. Professionals can also provide families with ideas for interacting through play at home. It is important to help parents understand that when they spend time playing with their children at home they are providing much needed support for their children in their grief. They are also building bonds that nurture their children's need for acceptance and bolsters their self-esteem.

Sometimes "Acting Out" Is How They Express Intense Emotions of Grief

It is difficult for children to understand and navigate the many intense emotions that accompany grief. Many of these feelings and reactions lack a language for expression. Because of this, it is normal for children to "act out" or for grief to find expression in ways that might be outside of what is socially acceptable. Many children we have provided support to over the years came to our programs with an attention deficit hyperactivity disorder (ADHD) diagnosis because of their behavior after a significant death in their life.

Too often, "acting out" is misunderstood in grieving children and, therefore, is misdiagnosed and treated with punishment, or in the case of ADHD, with medication. It is normal protocol for mental health and health care professionals assessing children with problem behaviors to do a complete history. This history should include questions about death, dying, and bereavement. If problem behaviors have occurred in close proximity to a significant loss, this information should be taken into consideration when recommending a course of action. Grieving children do not need to be "treated." Rather, they and their families can benefit from support and education. Support offers an understanding, caring environment to express their grief and education offers information and insight into why they are feeling the way they do.

If you are providing support to a bereaved child, consider the other adults in their lives and provide helpful information to them about how grief impacts the life of a child. It is also useful to share information with the child's parent, teachers, and other adults about how to maintain discipline while also acknowledging a child's grief. This information is provided to you in Chapter 4, in the section, "Affirming and Maintaining Boundaries."

They Often Feel Guilty

Children, especially younger children, see themselves as the center of their world. They are prone to magical thinking and often believe that good things and bad things happen in their lives because of their good and bad behaviors. Children will frequently express guilt after the death of someone in their lives, believing that had they been better behaved, or loved the person more, the person would not have died. This feeling is not always expressed and many children will carry this burden as they grow and develop. It is natural for children to retreat to a sense that they have some sort of control over their world particularly when dealing with the death of someone in their life, which can rob individuals of their sense of control. In this way, guilt can serve a purpose in reestablishing a sense of control and a sense that our choices matter. On the other hand, feeling as though they caused that person to die can also impact the way a child sees himself or herself.

Professionals can support children through this experience of guilt by providing opportunities to express these feelings free from judgment in the same way a child might express sadness, anger, or fear. Normalizing feelings of guilt can help children recognize that they are not the only ones feeling these as though the death is their fault. As children are able to openly express their thoughts and feelings in a safe way, they often find growth, insight, and support that helps them with feelings of guilt.

If You Don't Know What They Need From You, Just Ask

Many grieving children go without support simply because the adults in their lives do not know how to help them and are afraid that if they bring up the death it will make things worse. This happens far too often in the lives of bereaved children. It is okay to ask children their thoughts about the death. They will tell you if they want to talk about it or not. If they do not want to talk about it with you, they will tell you that. It is also okay for the adults in children's lives to ask them what they need from them during this time. With younger children it is helpful if you explain what that means. You can give them examples of what help might look like.

For example, a teacher might say privately to a newly bereaved child returning to school, "Your mother shared with me about what happened recently in your family with your father dying. I want you to know that we care about you and your family and that we want to be a help to you as you return to school. Please let me know when you need my help. An example of this might be if you are feeling sad and feel like you want to express that, I can give you a pass to go to see the school counselor for a little while." Grieving children are already thinking about the person who has died. They will let you know if they would rather not talk about or express it at that moment.

WHAT BEREAVED CHILDREN NEED

Honesty

Sharing the truth about how someone died can be difficult for the adults in children's lives. They often fear that knowing the truth will do more damage, so they look for ways to soften the truth or sometimes even avoid the truth altogether. As discussed in Chapter 3, in the section, "Share the Truth and Encourage Families to Do the Same," we outline reasons why telling the truth is important and why the language we use for discussing death with children is critical. Honesty is important with children to build trusting relationships with those caring for them. Grieving children will face many challenges along the way as they grow and develop. They are more likely to navigate this difficult journey with the trusted adults in their lives. Being dishonest with children early on in their grief can compromise these important relationships.

Reassurance

Grief can often be a lonely, difficult experience for children. As previously mentioned, children will grieve throughout their lives as they grow and develop. Children benefit from reassurance that they can continue to live their lives and thrive, even though someone in their life has died. It is important to educate the adults in children's lives that they have the ability to provide reassurance to children along the way. For example, Kassandra was 16 when her mother died from a long battle with cancer. Her father had left the family years prior to the death and Kassandra had to go live with her grandmother. During her senior year in high school, she struggled, as many young people do, with fear about leaving home and going to college. But she also had the added challenge of feeling like she was "alone" in this important transition and expressed that she "wished that her mother was here to help her through it."

Children need people in their lives to stand in this gap and provide the reassurance that they need along the way. Sometimes the simplest of tasks can seem hugely overwhelming to grieving children. A word of encouragement or support to work through problems or life situations can provide the reassurance they need and boost their confidence. Positive self-esteem is an important factor in promoting health in grieving children and can be bolstered by supportive, encouraging adults in children's lives.

Normalization

Grieving children benefit from knowing that a wide range of possible reactions to grief are normal. Children might feel confused by their own thoughts and feelings after a death. Most often, they lack a context for understanding these thoughts and feelings and will struggle to adapt them into their present reality. It is helpful when children interact with others going through a similar situation because often other grieving children are able to normalize some of these thoughts and feelings. Children can also normalize their thoughts and feelings by reading about other children going through similar situations.

Professionals can also use popular figures, both real and fantasy, to help children to normalize their thoughts, feelings, and situation. For example, almost all of the main characters in popular fairy tales, or super hero movies are bereaved children. Think of your favorite characters and try to think of one who is not bereaved. In the same way, many role models to children were bereaved as children as well. Professionals can share some of these individuals' stories with children, which will help to normalize their situation.

Validation

Akin to normalization, validation of a child's experience in grief is important. Validation of grief reactions happens when adults or peers in a child's life acknowledge what the child is feeling and allow the child the space needed to express his or her grief in the way that feels most natural to the child. Although it is important for the child to feel like he or she is not the only person experiencing grief, it is also important that the child is understood by the people closest to the child. Children will often look to their immediate caregiver for validation by seeking their attention. Think about a small child shouting out to a parent every few minutes, "Watch this!" The child is seeking validation from the parent that the child is important to the parent and that the parent is proud of the child's abilities. Grieving children need the adults in their lives to notice them, including how grief has impacted their lives.

SUMMARY

It is important for professionals to recognize the impact that grief has on the lives of children. Understanding the common reactions children have to grief and the factors that influence their grief enables the professional to better provide a safe environment for children to participate in support and counseling. It is essential to keep in mind that generalizations about children's grief should be approached as a way of understanding how grief might impact the lives of children. Caution should be used in applying these characterizations universally, however. Support professionals should always remember the Five Universal Realities of Grief and approach children as learners in the support and counseling setting.

REFERENCES

Andrews, C. R., & Marotta, S. A. (2005). Spirituality and coping among bereaved children: A preliminary study. *Counseling and Values, 50,* 38–50.

Bowlby, J. (1980). *Attachment and loss: Loss, sadness, and depression* (Vol. 3). New York, NY: Basic Books.

Corr, C. A., & Corr, D. M. (Eds.). (1996). *Handbook of childhood death and bereavement.* New York, NY: Springer Publishing.

DeSpelder, L. A., & Strickland, A. L. (2015). *The last dance: Encountering death and dying.* New York, NY: McGraw-Hill.

Gilbert, K., & Murray, C. (2007). The family, larger systems, and death education. In D. Balk, G. Thornton, & D. Meagher (Eds.), *Handbook of thanatology: The essential body of knowledge for the study of death, dying, and bereavement* (pp. 345–353). Northbrook, IL: The Association for Death Education and Counseling.

Kastenbaum, R. (2000). The kingdom where nobody dies. In K. J. Doka (Ed.), *Living with grief: Children, adolescents, and loss* (pp. 5–20). Washington, DC: Hospice Foundation of America.

Mahon, M. M. (1999). Secondary losses in bereaved children when both parents have died: A case study. *Omega—Journal of Death and Dying, 39,* 297–314.

McNiel, A., & Schuurman, D. L. (2016). Supporting grieving children. In B. P. Black, P. M. Wright, & R. Limbo (Eds.), *Perinatal and pediatric bereavement* (pp. 327–343). New York, NY: Springer Publishing.

Packman, W., Horsley, H., Davies, B., & Kramer, R. (2006). Sibling bereavement and continuing bonds. *Death Studies, 30,* 817–841.

Parkes, C. M., Laungani, P., & Young, W. (2015). *Death and bereavement across cultures.* New York, NY: Routledge.

Rando, T. A. (1993). *Treatment of complicated mourning.* Champaign, IL: Research Press.

Schoenfelder, E. N., Sandler, I. N., Wolchik, S., & MacKinnon, D. (2011). Quality of social relationships and the development of depression in parentally-bereaved youth. *Journal of Youth and Adolescence, 40,* 85–96.

Silverman, P. R., Baker, J., Cait, C., & Boerner, K. (2002–2003). The effects of negative legacies on the adjustment of parentally bereaved children and adolescents. *Omega—Journal of Death and Dying, 46,* 335–352.

Silverman, P. R., & Worden, J. W. (1992). Children's reactions in the early months after the death of a parent. *American Journal of Orthopsychiatry, 62,* 93–104.

Walsh, F., & McGoldrick, M. (Eds.). (2004). *Living beyond loss: Death in the family.* New York, NY: W. W. Norton.

Worden, J. W. (1996). *Children and grief: When a parent dies.* New York, NY: Guilford Press.

CHAPTER 3

Suicide, Homicide, Sudden Death, and Illness

I am thoroughly convinced that the most important, foundational, and critical need for bereaved children and teens is to feel understood, to know "I am not alone."

—*Donna Schuurman*

Similar to other factors that impact a child's grief, the cause of death can also influence a child's grief experience. Because of this there are special considerations that professionals should be aware of related to how a person died. The type of death has implications on each of the areas already discussed, from family dynamics after the death to the parent–child adaptive tasks. In this chapter, we explore specific types of death (suicide, homicide, sudden death, and illness) and how the potential circumstances surrounding these types of deaths influence a child's grief. In addition, this chapter provides professionals with information to better understand the impact on and reactions of children to each of these types of deaths.

DEATH BY SUICIDE

The grief experience following a death by suicide may be distressing for children in a way that is different from grief resulting from other causes of death (Cerel & Aldrich, 2011). After a suicide, children and families often feel shocked, blindsided, and dumbfounded. Many times, there is a sense of disbelief that the person died in this way and did this to the child or family. There is also confusion that someone they love would no longer want to be here. Children might wonder, "If my mom was feeling so upset, why wouldn't she ask me for help?" Suicide impacts a child's sense that the world is safe and predictable. Adding to the pain of suicide is the fact that, historically, these deaths have been stigmatized. Many of these stigmas continue today, making the grief experience even more difficult.

Reactions and Surrounding Circumstances

Hindsight Bias

Prior to dying, some individuals will directly express suicidal ideation. Other individuals might not come out and state that they want to die, but instead, might leave clues. After someone dies by suicide, family members often look back and try to piece together what happened. In this process of looking back, family members search for answers that are, most often, hard to find. Looking back can lead to hindsight bias. Hindsight bias can cause adults and children to feel guilty because they feel like they should have known what their loved ones were thinking about so that they could have stopped them. In fact, hindsight bias can cause family members to overestimate the probability of their ability to predict that a loved one would harm himself or herself (Goggin & Range, 1985).

Asking Why

Children might wonder why their person did not want to live anymore. It is difficult for children who have their entire lives in front of them to fully understand why a person would want to end his or her own life. Similarly, children might wonder how the person could harm himself or herself. It is hard for children to imagine hurting themselves, and they struggle with the idea that someone they love could do that to himself or herself.

Further, because children are egocentric and tend to view themselves as the center of the world, they will often take offense that the person did not think of them and how the suicide would impact their lives. A child might see it as a personal offense that the person would do this to the child. Children might wonder why the person would want to leave them, feeling as though the person did not love them enough to stay alive and be with them. For example, after Sarah's mother died, Sarah said, "If she loved me, she would not have left me." The unending questions and the question of "why" can be unrelenting for children and adults (Figure 3.1).

Blame

Sometimes children blame the person who died for taking his or her own life. This is related to their sense of anger over the person doing this to himself

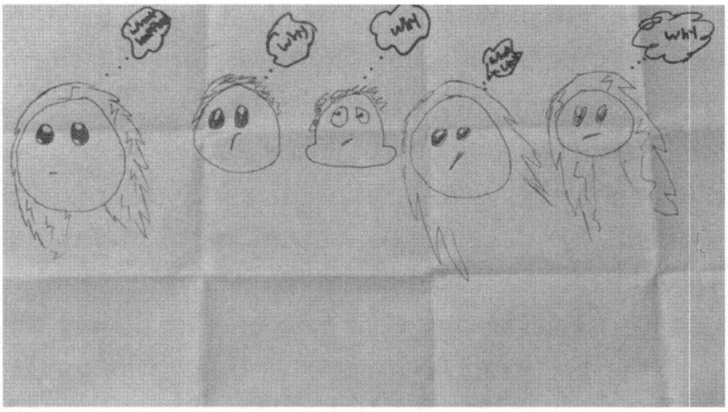

Figure 3.1 Artwork created by a preteen whose dad died.

or herself. For example, Melanie had a particularly close bond with her middle brother. They spent many hours playing together and talking about their lives together. After his death by suicide, she expressed, "I get so mad when I think about my brother doing this to himself. I just cannot understand why he would want to kill himself."

Children also sometimes blame other adults in their lives for not saving the person who died. For example, when Molly's father moved out after years of fighting and turmoil in the home, Molly blamed her mother for her father's moving out. When Molly's father later died from suicide, Molly was extremely angry with her mother and blamed her for her father's death. On one occasion she said to her mother, "Why did you make Dad leave? If you wouldn't have kicked him out, he would still be alive."

In other circumstances, children might blame a professional (e.g., doctor, psychologist, therapist) who was caring for a loved one for not saving him or her. Derrick's dad was going to the doctor because of depression. When Derrick's dad died from suicide, Derrick blamed his dad's doctor for not knowing that his dad was feeling suicidal and for not saving his father. On occasion, children will also blame themselves for the person's suicide. Sometimes children wonder whether if they had been nicer, more well behaved, or better people it would have prevented the suicide. Children also wonder what they could have done to save the person before the person ended his or her life.

Shame

According to Cerel, Fristad, Weller, and Weller (1999), children bereaved by suicide are more likely to experience anger, anxiety, and shame. Because of the societal stigma that is associated with suicide, children will often feel a sense of shame that their person died in this way. Because of this, some families will choose not to disclose that their relative died from suicide. Children will often follow the lead of their family and try to hide the way the person died from other people. It is important, however, that adults tell children the truth and strive to model being open about the true cause of death. When adults use the word *suicide*, even with younger children, this helps to destigmatize suicide and provides a truthful foundation on which to have further conversations, as children formulate more questions about the death. This helps children feel comfortable asking questions and receiving honest answers about what happened (Mitchell et al., 2006).

Another one of the unfortunate misconceptions and social stigmas about suicide is that it is a cowardly and selfish act. Because of this, sometimes children feel shame. Similar to messages that suicide is a sin, children tend to hear this message at school, in the community, and also in their own homes. This causes a sense of shame in children that the person was somehow a weak person. This thought might be in stark contrast to a child's elevated idea of who the person was.

Children might feel shame because of another social stigma, that suicide is a sin. There might be strongly held religious beliefs in their school, community, or home that perpetuate this notion. Children who hear these types of messages struggle with reconciling what this means in regard to the person's eternal fate. Messages such as these can cause further anger at the person who died and further complicate a child's adjustment to the reality of the loss and the changes this brings to the child's life.

Worry

As with other types of loss, children whose person died from suicide may worry about a number of things. Children might wonder whether suicide is hereditary and that it might happen to someone else in their family. This might cause them to worry about their own future and whether they will have the same struggle as the person who died. They might also worry about who else in their life might die, causing them to become overly protective of the surviving adults in their family.

DEATH BY HOMICIDE

Death resulting from violence or homicide leaves a lasting impact on families (Currier, Holland, Coleman, & Neimeyer, 2008). After a homicide, family members often feel as though the world is cruel and unjust (DeSpelder & Strickland, 2015) and in the wake of a homicide, families typically experience a tremendous amount of anxiety, stress, fear, and sadness. This is a result of the often violent, public, and sudden nature of homicide. Another aspect of a homicide is that there might be ongoing legal or court proceedings. The trial and sentencing process can take months or even years to resolve, directing family attention and energy toward a desire for justice. This can sometimes delay grief until after a case is completed. If the perpetrator is captured and found guilty, children and their family members might feel that it is not enough punishment to compensate for their loss. Sometimes individuals worry about their own safety or the safety of others after a homicide (Bordere, 2014). Another pervasive feeling that children might have is whether they could have done anything to change the outcome.

Often, homicides attract media attention. In high-profile cases, a family might feel exposed and exploited by the media. As a result, children might experience a sense of loss of control over their own lives. In addition, families sometimes lose their support system after a homicide. One of the reasons for this is that people often don't know what to say, or they are worried that they might say the wrong thing, so they don't say anything at all. In addition to these types of impact, children also experience a number of reactions to a homicide that are unique to this type of loss.

Reactions and Surrounding Circumstances

Fear

After a homicide, children may experience fear for their own safety. The death of a family member by homicide can heighten the natural tendency of children to experience fear. Children might be afraid that they, too, will be murdered by the perpetrator, particularly if the person has not been caught. Even if the perpetrator has been caught, children can still be afraid of being harmed. In addition to fearing for themselves, children may also experience fear for the safety of other family members. Children grieving a death by homicide have a heightened sense that people can perpetrate horrific violence against one another. If the person was murdered by another family member or someone the victim knew, this further reinforces a child's fear about the safety of other family members.

For example, Nathan was in the car with two other friends when two gunmen shot up the car they were in. Both of Nathan's friends were killed, but Nathan was able to work his way onto the floor board of the car and survive. It had been almost a year since the shooting, but the two gunmen were never identified or arrested. Nathan was terrified to leave his house in fear that the gunmen knew who he was and would come after him.

Rage

As previously mentioned, anger is a common grief reaction in children after someone dies. After a death by homicide, anger is often intensified and expressed in terms of rage. Rage is a mounting, violent type of anger that is sparked by a homicide. Children might become enraged or experience strong feelings of wanting to hurt the person who perpetrated the homicide. This might manifest itself in the form of fantasies or "daydreams" of these types of actions. This is not to be confused with revenge, which is associated with justice and forethought. This form of rage is associated with intense anger toward the person who committed the crime.

Children might also experience an overall sense of feeling enraged or a heighted sense of aggression. This could be directed at people in general or situations in general and could lead to a lack of patience or tolerance for other people. Children experiencing this type of rage often have a hard time caring about anything, including school, friends, and family. In most instances, rage is not a long-term reaction, but tends to de-escalate or diminish with a combination of time, family support, and perspective.

Revenge

The desire to take matters into your own hands and seek revenge is related to justice. Revenge is similar to rage, in which a person might want to harm the perpetrator. The difference is that revenge tends to involve plotting or planning. This is a common reaction to homicide, often born out as a fantasy. Children do not typically enact their fantasies of revenge, although exceptions would be in cases of gang violence or "street justice." It is important to note that revenge could be motivated by a sense of rage.

Children will often imagine scenarios in which the person who committed the crime is "getting what he deserves." They may or may not fantasize about enacting what they perceive to be justice on the person themselves. Sometimes children and other family members place high expectations on court proceedings. When the court proceedings are slow or do not deliver the desired results, children and their families might experience frustration with the judicial system.

Thoughts of Revenge

It is not unusual for feelings of revenge to seep into the thoughts of children after a homicide. Sometimes these thoughts will reflect sentiments of revenge held by their adult caregivers. Often adults who have a stronger desire for revenge have an equally strong desire for justice and are overly concerned with the court proceedings. Children could be negatively impacted if they have a caregiver who is expressing a desire for revenge.

SUDDEN DEATH

Sudden deaths may also produce distinct reactions in children. Examples of sudden death are heart attacks, strokes, and car accidents. Sudden deaths are often characterized by a sense of shock and disbelief that the person was here one moment and then gone the next (Silverman & Worden, 1992). Many children bereaved after a sudden death report feeling like they were in a fog and that they could not believe that the person was really dead. Because of the suddenness of the death, younger children might feel as though the person has just gone on a long trip and is not really dead. In fact, in this case, younger children might be expecting the deceased to return home at any time.

Reactions and Surrounding Circumstances

Regret

In cases of sudden death, bereaved children often feel a sense of regret. Typically regret is the result of wanting the opportunity to do or say something differently. Children might regret that they did not get to say goodbye. This is a common reaction surrounding many types of sudden deaths. By the very nature of the death being sudden and unexpected, people often express, "When he left the house this morning, I never expected it to be the last time I would see him alive."

Children might also ruminate over conversations and interactions with the person who died. It is not uncommon for children to have feelings of regret for things they said or did not say, or for their last interaction with the person who died. This is particularly true when the conversation or interaction was confrontational, argumentative, or negative in any way. For example, children might express regret over an argument in which mean words were exchanged, particularly if this were their last interaction with the person who died.

Not only will children ruminate over conversations and last interactions, they may also be very hard on themselves for negative thoughts they might have had about the person prior to the person's death. This can lead to intense feelings of regret. For example, a child being punished by a parent might think in their mind, "I hate you and wish you were dead." Then Dad dies suddenly and the child struggles with regret over his thoughts.

Guilt

In certain circumstances of sudden death, children might feel guilty about their role in the person's death. This guilt can be real or imagined, but either way it is experienced as an authentic feeling about what has happened. For example, sometimes children feel guilty as a result of being directly responsible for the death of another person. An unfortunate, but common, example of this is a teenage driver of a car that crashes and kills some of the teen's friends. Being the driver of the car in an instance like this produces strong feelings of guilt and personal responsibility in the driver of the car.

Another example is when a child accidentally shoots a friend or family member; it is common for the child to experience feelings of intense guilt, even when the child knows it was unintentional. Children feel a sense of guilt over the death of someone even when they were not directly responsible. This could be a situation in which the child witnessed the death and felt like he or she could have done something to prevent it. Children can also have these feelings even when they were not present for the death.

Children might also have a sense of guilt that something they did or said set things in motion that led to someone's death. For example, Jamal asked his dad to come to his basketball game. His dad left work early to get to the game on time, but died in a car accident on the way. Jamal felt personally responsible for his dad's death because he asked him to come to the basketball game. He felt like his dad would still be alive had he not asked him to leave work early and come to the game. This type of imagined guilt is associated with believing that the child had the power to change the outcome.

Anger

Anger is an emotion that is common to a variety of types of losses. Sudden losses, however, evoke feelings of anger unique to the circumstances of the sudden loss (a car accident, heart attack, etc.). Children might experience anger at the person who died for not taking care of his or her health. They might be angry at someone because the person smoked, or didn't eat healthfully and had medical conditions as a result. For example, Rachel would constantly fuss at her dad for smoking. When her dad died of a heart attack associated with pulmonary disease, she could not help feeling angry at her dad for smoking and blamed him for what happened.

Similarly, children might experience anger at the person who died for being careless. For example, Mike's brother was always behaving recklessly with his friends. They would dare each other to do stunts and other "daredevil" types of things. His friends dared him to jump off one of the local bridges into the water and swim to shore. He jumped and never surfaced. Mike experienced extreme anger toward his brother for being careless and, in Mike's mind, causing his own death.

DEATH FROM ILLNESS

There are certain reactions to death resulting from an illness that are particular to this type of loss. A family's journey with the illness and ultimately the impending death of a family member contribute to these reactions. For example, if the illness was long term, children and families experience a number of challenges and losses along the way as the illness progresses and the ill person's physical health worsens. During this time, children may or may not play a role in the daily care of the person. Some families will attempt to shield children from the harsh realities of the illness, whereas others share the condition openly with the children. Quite often, when children are not given information about the illness, they feel blindsided when the illness ultimately leads to death. In this case, children will often feel resentment toward their caregivers for not sharing information with them or including them in the details of the illness. The following are additional reactions and surrounding circumstances that are common to grief over death resulting from an illness.

Important Considerations Leading Up to a Death Resulting From Illness

In the same way that the death of a family member impacts the dynamics within the family unit, so do long-term, life-limiting, terminal illnesses. There are factors that warrant further consideration in regard to children anticipating the death of someone in their lives. Just because a death resulting from illness is anticipated, this does not mean that children will necessarily adjust more easily than a death that was not anticipated (Saldinger, Cain, Kalter, & Lognes, 1999). The terminal illness of a close family member affects the day-to-day lives of children. Parents and caregivers sometimes struggle with what to share, how much to share, and when to share information about what is happening with their children.

Dealing With the Diagnosis

Typically, parents will grapple with the enormity of a diagnosis themselves even before considering what to tell the children. Depending on who has been diagnosed—one of the parents, a child in the family, or a grandparent—this process of dealing with the diagnosis could take much time. During this time, children will often overhear conversations, or learn what is going on from other family members. In other cases, children might sense changes in their parents' moods, and slight shifts in family dynamics. Professionals should be patient with parents as they work through their own reactions to the diagnosis, while also advocating for the best interest of the children. Each family might approach the diagnosis and how to involve the children in different ways. Although there is no cookie-cutter approach to talking with children about death, there are some important considerations that have implications on the health of children throughout the illness and process of dying of a family member.

Telling the Children

Parents often do not know how to talk to their child when there's a terminal illness or how to prepare them for the person's eventual death. Because of this, children are often left in the dark about what is happening with the person who is sick. Parents and caregivers are often scared to tell children the truth about what is happening. This is typically well-meaning, as they are trying to preserve their child's innocence and protect him or her from a harsh reality about life. The problem is that children are more often than not aware of what is going on around them or aware that they're not being told everything (Sweder, 1995). They notice if adults stop talking as they enter the room. They notice if adults seem sad or stressed. They notice body language. The best approach is for professionals to suggest to parents to make a plan for when, what, and how to tell the children about the illness and the implications that the illness of a loved one will have on the family. If children are not told, they are left to question and wonder on their own without help from the adults around them.

When to Tell the Children

When to tell the children is an important consideration. Sometimes families have limited information themselves about the illness and might want to hold off telling the children until they have more concrete information. However, it is often best to tell the children as soon as possible because a lack of knowledge about what is happening can cause stress in children. It is important for children to be included in end-of-life conversations so that they will not be forced to handle this by themselves (Robinson, 2012). Children cope better when they are included in conversations about the illness and care of a loved one (DeSpelder & Strickland, 2015). This does not mean that the moment someone is diagnosed with a long-term or terminal illness, you immediately start discussing death with children. Timing is important.

There are new treatments every day for different types of terminal conditions and many people live for many years with different types of illnesses.

However, opening communication with children from the beginning provides a context for children to feel like they are part of the family, that their feelings matter, and that they can ask questions along the way. So professionals should encourage families to provide factual information about the illness, the treatment, how the treatment will affect the ill person, and how the family will need to help out at the time of diagnosis. Professionals should also encourage parents to share information and updates along the way, and to make themselves available to their child to answer any questions they might have.

When the prognosis is that the illness will lead to death and that treatments are no longer effective, it might take some time for the patient and a child's parents to deal with this reality. Again, professionals should be patient with families as they wrestle with this difficult reality. At the same time, professionals can provide helpful information to families about how to transition the conversation from treatment to preparing for the death of a family member. There are many things that families can do to make the most of the time they have with the person who is dying when everyone in the family is on the same page.

How to Tell the Children

Professionals should encourage parents to consider the setting when discussing the illness or impending death with their children. Preferably, a quiet setting with trusted relatives in the room or nearby is best. It is ideal if it is a parent or other trusted adult who is sharing the information, rather than a professional (Marshall, Manning, & Mercer, 2013). This option should be exhausted first before a professional considers delivering this information to children. Allowing the parents or another trusted family member to share the information with the children lays a foundation for future communication and trust. This will help children know where to direct their questions along the way as well.

Some parents tell all of the children at the same time, whereas others tell the kids at different times depending on their age. Some parents opt to tell older children and teenagers first, but it is important to remember not to exclude young children. Information shared should be age appropriate, depending on the developmental age of a child. Younger children will need information in "bite-sized" pieces so that they have time to process the information (this could happen over a series of days or even weeks).

Professionals should advise parents to encourage children to ask questions about things they don't understand. For example, "Is there anything that I've told you that you're wondering about?" or "Is there anything that I've told you that you have a question about?" Presenting the information in a calm, loving, direct manner will help to establish open communication lines with children.

What if a Parent Is Adamant That the Children Do Not Need to Know?

This is an important question to address, as you are likely to encounter families who are convinced that they can protect children from the harsh reality of the illness. First and foremost, it is important for a professional in this scenario to avoid being judgmental of the family's ideas. It is always helpful to begin by trying to understand the family's perspective or thoughts about the matter. Most often families believe they are protecting their children and working in their best interest. When they feel heard by you, this can open doors to further communication on the subject. When a trusting, mutually respectful relationship has been established, there are some helpful questions you might pose to the family for their consideration. These questions are detailed in the section "Share the Truth and Encourage Families to Do the Same."

What to Tell the Children

Parents should be encouraged that children need to know the truth and that it can be provided incrementally with age-appropriate detail. A good first step to suggest to parents is for them to ask the children what they've been observing and what they think is happening or what changes have they noticed (in the ill family member or in the family as a whole). Even if they do not have much to say, providing information in a conversational manner opens the door for ongoing dialogue.

Then, encourage parents to explain to the children what is happening. Encourage the parents to attempt to give the children information using language that they can understand. Parents should expect that there might be a lot of questions (though this is not the case with every child).

When it comes to discussing treatment, it's important to explain what treatment means. If treatment has changed from what the child has previously been told, it is important to explain that the treatment has changed. Any time a new term is introduced to a child, a parent should do his or her best to define that term in a way the child can understand. Encourage parents to use the name of the illness when talking with the children. For example, it is important for children to understand that cancer is different from a cold or the flu. Children often worry about others when they are sick or even worry about themselves and can sometimes associate illnesses that are not life-threatening with those that are.

When the appropriate time comes to discuss a person's death with the child, professionals should encourage parents to use clear, concrete language. Parents should avoid euphemisms such as *passing away* or *going to sleep*. It is appropriate for parents to explain the death in the context of their religious beliefs, but they should be encouraged to use words like *die* or *death* to describe the physical process that is taking place. It is confusing to children, particularly younger children, when they are told someone is going to heaven without understanding that the person's body is dying.

For example, a dad took his 4-year-old daughter to his grandmother's funeral. There was an open casket for viewing and he walked up to the casket holding his daughter in his arms. Dad shared a few memories about his grandmother with his daughter and then they returned to their seats to wait for the service to begin. A couple of minutes after they sat down, his daughter looked up at him and said, "Dad, I thought you said grandmamma was in heaven?" To which he replied, "Well, sweetie, she is in heaven." To which she replied, "Well, if grandmamma is in heaven, who is that in that box up there?"

It is helpful for children to hear language that is clear about death and dying. As mentioned earlier, younger children struggle with understanding fully what it means to be dead, so being clear with them will help as they come to understand what death means.

Reactions and Circumstances Surrounding a Death Caused by Illness

Relief

It is difficult for children and families to watch a person they love suffer. Individuals often report feeling a sense of helplessness when watching someone suffer pain from an illness. Because of this, it is common for children grieving a death from illness to feel a sense of relief that the person is no longer in pain and that they do not have to see them suffering any longer. In a similar way, children might feel relief if the person was sick for a long time. This is particularly true if the child was assigned responsibilities to help take care of the person.

When there is a lengthy illness, the illness becomes an integral, yet draining, part of the home environment and family dynamics. Providing care to a person who is sick takes a large amount of time and energy. Also, having a sick person in the home can sometimes interrupt children's lives; for example, it may prevent them from inviting friends over to play or spend the night. Children can sometimes resent the person who is sick because of this and express relief when the person dies and the home returns to a more normal environment.

Guilt

Children sometimes experience guilt because they avoided spending time with the sick person. This reluctance can be caused by a number of reasons. There are many aspects of illness that are difficult for children to witness. These can include the physical deterioration of someone they love, the intense suffering that is sometimes associated with illnesses, or the high level of personal care often required by the ill person. Children might avoid spending time with the person because of the overwhelming nature of the situation, and then later feel guilty.

Many children who seek counseling under our care have also reported feelings of guilt because of their sense of relief after the death. These concurrent feelings are common, particularly when the illness was lengthy or the person who was sick experienced much suffering.

Regret

Children will often report feelings of regret after someone dies from an illness. An important distinction needs to be made between guilt and regret, as discussed in Chapter 1. If children feel like they made personal choices that caused them to miss time and opportunities to be with the person who was sick, this is most often expressed as guilt. If children wished they could have had more time with the person, but do not necessarily express that they avoided time with the person intentionally, then that is more likely a sense of regret rather than guilt.

Sometimes children will express that they wish they had been able to do more for the person who was sick. This includes relieving the person's pain or providing some type of care to bring the person more comfort. Often they are not sure what that would have been, but still feel a sense of regret for not being able to do more to help the sick person. This can also be related to feelings of helplessness they might have experienced when the person was still alive.

Children will also experience feelings of regret, wishing they could have had more time to spend with the person who was sick. For example, Jason regretted that he had so many school and after-school activities that took him away from time with his mother when she was sick. He reflected back and said, "If I would have known that she was going to die so soon from this, I would have been less involved with things at school and spent more time with her." Quite often in an effort to spare children from the harsh realities of a sickness, adults will not tell them someone is sick enough to die. Children will regret that they did not spend more time with the person and wish they had known the person was going to die (Figure 3.2).

Worry About Illnesses

Children who have had a person die from an illness will often become hypersensitive to their own illnesses and the illnesses of others, even when they are not life threatening. For example, a child whose parent died from cancer might worry when he or she has a cold that he or she also has cancer. The child might have these same worries about family members if the family members are exhibiting similar symptoms as the person who died.

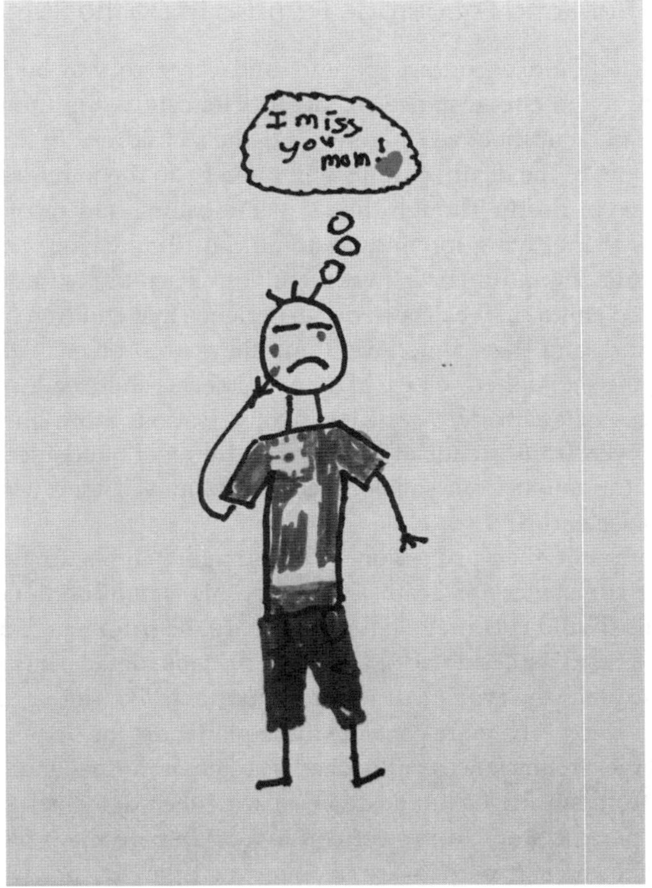

Figure 3.2 Artwork created by a teenager whose mom died.

How to Help

This section provides key principles for professionals about how to help bereaved children and their families, as well as special considerations that apply to certain circumstances of death. These principles apply across the board no matter the circumstances of the death, though there are some distinctions that are specific to certain causes of death. Understanding these principles will help the professional support the children under their care, and provide the parents or caregivers of children with the information they need to support their children.

Share the Truth and Encourage Families to Do the Same

Professionals should encourage parents and caregivers to be honest with children about the circumstances of death. Honesty is the foundation of a trusting relationship between parents and their children. In an attempt to soften the blow of the death, parents will often lie to their children about the circumstances of death. Though this is well-meaning and most of the time done out of caring, lying to children about the circumstances of death can lead to resentment and mistrust when children learn the truth. In our work with bereaved children, it has been our experience that children often already know the truth and they sometimes think they are protecting their parents by keeping the secret themselves. In other instances, children learn about the circumstances of death by overhearing conversations from another family member or even from friends at school. Children feel blindsided when they learn this information from someone else, especially if they were told a lie about the cause of death.

It is important that professionals encourage parents to tell the truth about the circumstances of death. However, this should be done with care. Professionals should encourage parents to share the truth in age-appropriate, bite-sized pieces. There is no need to share gruesome details, but using actual terms that explain the type of death are important, like *suicide, homicide, car accident*, and *cancer*. The more concrete the explanation, the better. Sharing the truth about the circumstances of the death is often more challenging when the death was from suicide or homicide because of the stigmas associated with both. Also, parents want to protect children and spare them from thinking about these realities. If parents are adamant that they do not want to share the truth with their child, there are a few questions you might pose as the professional to help parents feel more comfortable.

First, ask the parent, "Are you certain that your child does not already know?" This is an important first question because quite often they are not sure of this. If they say they are not sure, then you can move quickly to the next question. You then ask, "If it is possible that your child already knows the truth, then would you prefer he or she wrestles with the truth alone, or with you?" In our experience working with parents, this awareness that their child might be grappling with this difficult knowledge on his or her own is enough to convince parents to share the truth with their child no matter how difficult that truth might be.

If the parents, in reply to the first question, answers that they are certain that their child does not yet know the truth and that they are not going to tell them the truth, the professional can then follow up with one more question. The professional can ask, "Are you certain that your child will never know the truth about how this person died for the rest of his or her life? Can you guarantee your child will not learn the truth? If not, you are risking your child not trusting you to tell the truth should he or she find out somehow. You are also risking your child finding out and having to deal with this harsh reality on his or her own, rather than with you." Again, in our experience, when most parents ponder this final question and advice, they typically answer that they cannot guarantee that their child will never know the truth. Most of the time, parents will then seek information and support from the professional to share the truth with their child.

The professional can then explain to the parents how to share information with their child in an age-appropriate, honest way. Remind parents that younger children might need to be told multiple times as they might ask over and over again how the person died. Remind parents that they can begin simply by using the right words to talk about the death, like, "Dad died from suicide (or homicide, cancer, etc.)." Children will ask questions as they have them and parents can answer their questions honestly using caution not to overshare.

Model Accurate Language

Just as important as being honest with children is using accurate language when talking to children about a death. As previously mentioned, using the correct terms that refer to particular types of deaths, such as *suicide, homicide*, or *cancer*, are important so that children do not associate the death with anything other than the reality of how it happened. This also gives children a context for understanding how death happens. If instead of "cancer" the person is said to have died because she was "sick," it is not unusual for children to worry about the well-being of others in their family when they are sick with a cold because children do not have a context for understanding that cancer is different from a cold.

Very particular to the circumstance of a suicide is the language we use to describe this type of death. The common way to refer to suicide in our society is to say that someone *committed suicide*. This phrase is widely used by the media, therapists, physicians, and lay people alike. It is important to understand, though, that this phrase is offensive to many people, especially those grieving the suicide death of someone. The term *commit* harkens to a time when suicide was thought of as a crime, and in many religious communities was considered a sin that came with very specific punishment, including not being able to be buried with religious ceremonies or in sacred ground.

As we learn more about suicide today and what brings people to the place where they take their own lives, these archaic understandings of suicide must be challenged. One way to do this is to change the language we use when we talk about suicide. Rather than say someone *committed* suicide, we can instead use language similar to how we talk about other types of death. When someone dies from cancer, we say they died *from* cancer. When someone dies of a heart attack, we say they died *of* a heart attack. So, using this same language, we can say that someone died *from* suicide or *of* suicide. Died *by* suicide is also a term commonly used in place of *committed* suicide.

Though it is important to model accurate language, the professional should avoid imposing his or her language on families. We recommend sharing written information and resources that educate families about issues specific to certain circumstances of death, rather than correcting their language during support sessions. For example, many families bereaved by a suicide death will use the term *committed* suicide to describe what happened to the person who died. There is no need to correct a family's verbiage. Families can refer to their own grief in their own terms. It is enough to model accurate language and to educate other professionals to do the same.

Provide Information About Handling Stress

The experience of grief is stressful no matter the circumstances of death. However, some circumstances of death produce more stress than others because of the intensity and nature of the loss. Because of this, professionals should be prepared with information for children and families about how to cope with stress, as well as ways to destress in any given moment. One simple way to do this with children is to teach them some deep-breathing exercises by using visual images that require them to inhale and exhale deeply in a controlled manner. Deep breathing evokes a physical reaction that reduces stress in individuals, including children (Varvogli & Darviri, 2011).

The professional can engage children in a discussion about stress. It is optimal if they can get children to share what they think stress is and how stress impacts their life. They can then identify times when children feel stressed. Professionals can then teach children to do deep breathing by using the following simple technique. Ask children to imagine that they are holding a fragrant flower. Then tell children to breathe in through the nose deeply as if they are taking in the wonderful smell of the fragrant flower. Tell them to breathe in as much air as they can and then blow the air out of their mouths as if they are trying to blow the petals off of the flower. Instruct the children that they can do this type of deep breathing five or six times in a row in moments they are experiencing stress to relieve their feelings of stress.

Be Patient With Children and Their Families

We cannot emphasize enough how important it is to be patient with bereaved children and their families. Children move through and experience their grief at their own pace. It can be challenging at times for professionals to allow children to struggle with many of the intense feelings brought about by their grief. But it is important that they are allotted whatever time they need to grieve in the way that feels most comfortable to them. Quite often in the life of bereaved children, people are trying to hurry them through the painful feelings of grief to a place of happiness and resolve. This is, however, a mistake and does little to relieve the feelings children are experiencing. When encouraged to feel better, children will often stop showing these feelings, but this does not mean they are not experiencing them. Attempting to push children to "feel better" only leaves them to grieve alone. Remember, grief is not a problem we are trying to fix; it is an experience bereaved children are living.

This also applies to helping parents to share truthful and accurate information with their children. Once you have provided the information they need and discussed the importance of telling the truth with them, be patient with parents as they come to terms with the reality they are facing. Keep in mind that parents are grieving, too, and that they are experiencing an entirely new reality that has many unknowns, surprises, and challenges to navigate. They will need the support of others, including professionals, along the way. So, it is important to preserve the relationship by being patient with parents as they face their grief.

Provide Space for Children to Talk About the Death and Meet Them Where They Are

Quite often, children have a need to talk specifically about the death. This can include everything from why people have to die to the gruesome details of how someone died. It is important to allow space for this in the support setting and to ensure that children are not "shut down" if they are sharing this type of information. For many children there is a need to talk about the images of the death that are in their mind. As they are able to tell about these images, they are constructing a narrative about what has happened. They are also able to recall these images in a space that is safe and free from the intense emotions, or even chaos, that might have been occurring when they first were told about, or experienced, the death. Professionals might find that children will tell the same stories over and over again. This is common as children are attempting to accommodate their mental constructs about the world around them so they can adapt this tragic event into their understanding of how the world works.

Further, it is important when supporting bereaved children to "meet them where they are." This means that children will bring their own particular likes, dislikes, preferences, personalities, and experiences with them into the support setting. As previously discussed in Chapter 1, a child's grief belongs to the child, including the way the child feels supported in his or her grief. Professionals should pay attention to how children are responding to discussions and activities. They should follow the lead of the children they are supporting and allow the children to teach them (the professionals) where they are in their grief and what they find to be helpful.

Know Community Resources and Appropriate Referrals

Finally, it is important for professionals to be aware of community resources and appropriate referrals for children in regard to particular circumstances of death. As previously discussed in Chapter 1, when children are experiencing symptoms of trauma and those symptoms persist, professionals should determine whether a referral is appropriate to assess for post traumatic stress disorder. Helping parents find the right resources for their children is of the utmost importance.

Also, there are community organizations and support groups that are specific to particular circumstances of death. Many communities have victim's assistance programs for families of people who died by homicide. It can be helpful for families to connect with these resources as they will often need ongoing support through court proceedings and other legal implications that could drag on for some time after the death. In the case of suicide, there are groups across North America providing support specific to suicide. Referrals to these groups can be found through the American Foundation for Suicide Prevention.

SUMMARY

Homicide, suicide, sudden death, and illness all have specific implications on the lives of children and their families. Homicide and suicide are often stigmatized and leave children confused and wondering why the person died in this way. Although other types of sudden deaths do not typically have the same stigma as homicide and suicide, they can be marked by intensified reactions, such as anger and bewilderment. The death of a family member as the result of an illness also has specific implications on a child's grief. Professionals should consider how the person died when providing support to children who are grieving. This can provide insight into how grief might be manifesting itself in the child's life. Yet, as previously noted, children should be given the opportunity to express their own unique experiences within the support setting. Professionals should provide space for children to share their stories and characterize their grief in terms of their choosing.

REFERENCES

Bordere, T. C. (2014). Adolescents and homicide. In K. J. Doka & A. S. Tucci (Eds.), *Living with grief: Helping adolescents cope with loss.* Washington, DC: Hospice Foundation of America.

Cerel, J., & Aldrich, R. S. (2011). The impact of suicide children and adolescents. In J. R. Jordan & J. L. McIntosh (Eds.), *Grief after suicide: Understanding the consequences and caring for the survivors* (pp. 81–92). New York, NY: Routledge, Taylor & Francis Group.

Cerel, J., Fristad, M. A., Weller, E. B., & Weller, R. A. (1999). Suicide-bereaved children and adolescents: A controlled longitudinal examination. *Journal of the American Academy of Child & Adolescent Psychiatry, 38,* 672–679.

Currier, J. M., J. Holland, J. M., Coleman, R. A., & Neimeyer, R. A. (2008). Bereavement following violent death: An assault on life and meaning. In R. G. Stevenson & G. R. Cox (Eds.), *Perspectives on violence and violent deaths* (pp. 172–202). Amityville, NY: Bayville Publishing.

DeSpelder, L. A., & Strickland, A. L. (2015). *The last dance: Encountering death and dying.* New York, NY: McGraw-Hill.

Goggin, W. C., & Range, L. M. (1985). The disadvantages of hindsight in the perception of suicide. *Journal of Social and Clinical Psychology, 3,* 232–237.

Marshall, S., Manning, J., & Mercer, S (2013). Encouraging/supporting dying parents to talk to their children. *End of Life Journal, 3,* 1–4.

Mitchell, A. M., Wesner, S., Brownson, L., Gale, D. D., Garand, L., & Havill, A., (2006). Effective communication with bereaved child survivors of suicide. *Journal of Child and Adolescent Psychiatric Nursing, 19,* 130–136.

Robinson, V. (2012). Communication vignettes: Telling a child that her dad is dying. *End of Life Journal, 2,* 1–4.

Saldinger, A., Cain, A., Kalter, N., & Lognes, K. (1999). Anticipating parental death in families with young children. *Journal of Orthopyschiatry, 69,* 39–48.

Silverman, P. R., & Worden, J. W. (1992). Children's reactions in the early months after the death of a parent. *American Journal of Orthopsychiatry, 62,* 93–104.

Sweder, G. (1995). Talking to children about the terminal illness of a loved one. In E. A. Grollman (Ed.), *Bereaved children and teens: A support guide for parents and professionals* (pp. 47–59). Boston, MA: Beacon Press.

Varvogli, L., & Darviri, C. (2011). Stress management techniques: Evidence-based procedures that reduce stress and promote health. *Health Science Journal, 5,* 74–89.

CHAPTER 4

Death of a Parent

You are the bows from which your children as living arrows are sent forth.

—*Kahlil Gibran*, The Prophet

A CHILD'S CONCEPT OF A PARENT

Our understanding of the concept of a parent is one that evolves as we see ever-changing family structures. Today single-parent homes (Vespa, Lewis, & Kreider, 2013), grandparents and other family members raising children (Ellis & Simmons, 2014), and same-sex couples raising children are more commonplace (Lofquist, 2011). This backdrop is important to the discussion of a child adapting to the death of a parent because it is the child who defines who his or her parent is, not the social construct of a male and female partnership. This is perhaps the most important piece of information a professional needs to know from a child. Ideally, the parent provides love, stability, and guidance to his or her children. But this is not always the case, so professionals should allow children to lead them to an understanding of what their relationship with the deceased person was like. In this chapter, we explore how a child is impacted by and adapts to the death of a parental figure, and the challenges that brings to the relationship to the surviving parental figure (the person with primary caregiving duties in the life of the child following the death). This information provides professionals with information about how to help children and their surviving parent successfully navigate the Parent–Child Adaptive Tasks section, found later in this chapter, following the death of a parent (Figure 4.1).

THE DEATH OF A PARENT

The death of a parent is a life-altering experience at any age. For a child, the death of a parent is especially difficult and the impact of the death is

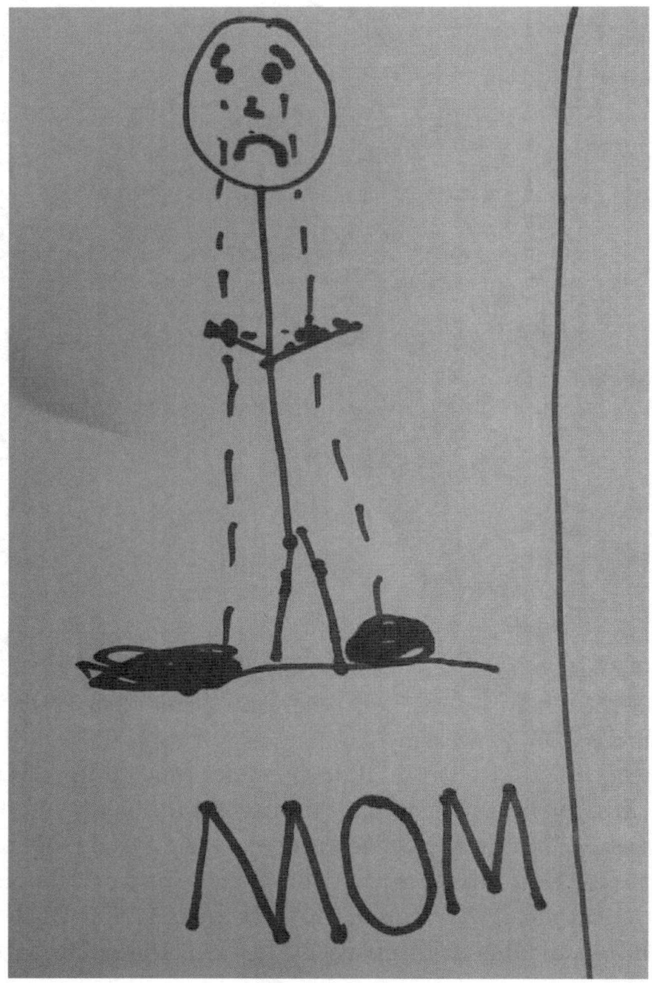

Figure 4.1 Artwork created by a younger child whose mom died.

often felt in every area of a child's life (Silverman & Worden, 1992). This, of course, is dependent on the child's relationship with the deceased parent. In many homes, when a parent dies, young children are deprived of the love, stability, and guidance that the parent would have potentially provided, as well as the long-term sense of security that the parent would have offered. Children depend on their parents to meet a variety of needs, some more obvious than others. In other homes, the death of a parent might bring about more stability, particularly when children are dealing with difficult situations with a parent such as addiction, abandonment, or abuse. It is important that professionals provide space for children to share about their experiences and express their sentiment about what the death of this person means to them (Figure 4.2).

STRENGTHS OF THE PARENT–CHILD RELATIONSHIP IMPACTED BY GRIEF

Just as there are a variety of family structures, there are also a variety of circumstances and situations that might define children's relationships with their primary caregiver. In the ideal situation, a parent provides love, stability, and guidance. When discussing the strengths of a parent–child relationship, we should recognize that, in many ways, we are discussing the best-case situation. Many children are dealing with difficult relationships with their parents, including alcoholism, drug addiction, abandonment, or abuse. Sometimes children might even feel relieved after a parent's death in some of these types of situations because their environment improves in the absence of the deceased. Yet, even in situations in which there was dysfunction of some type, it is also common for children to have conflicting emotions. "I love my dad, but I hated when he would drink and yell at us." The suggestions given in this chapter are effective approaches to helping children and their surviving parent adapt to the changes that death brings to the family. They provide a context for helping a family organize their environment and relationships after a death. Suggestions given here should be adapted to address the variety of circumstances encountered when working with children and their families.

Social Cues and Problem Solving

Parents typically provide children with information about the world, from social cues to solving problems. Children learn to interact with others their

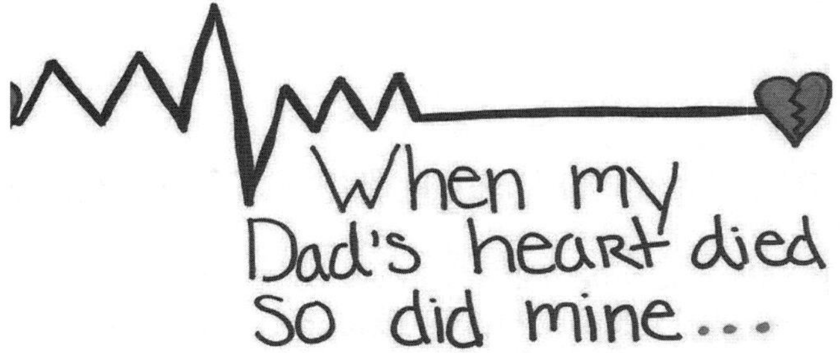

Figure 4.2 Artwork created by a teenager whose dad died.

own age and look to their parents to model appropriate behaviors when dealing with peers. Parents are often there with their children when they are learning about how the world works and to answer their many questions about the mysteries of life. Though children learn many facts and figures at school, their parents are the ultimate teachers in the home (good or bad), providing important information that is steeped in culture and traditional stories that help to frame the way children see the world.

Security and Predictability

Parents provide their children with a sense of security and predictability. In many instances, families function within daily routines, traditions, and predictable interactions that serve as stabilizers in children's lives. Children learn that even when their parents go away, they come back. They come to expect certain behaviors from their parents as they learn to navigate the boundaries of the home environment and expectations set by their parents. As they grow and develop, these routines become a part of their understanding of how the world works. This impact is felt by the child both in the short term and the long term. Immediately after a loss, children's daily routines are impacted and changes are felt. The impact on their routine could be anything from who will now take them to school in the morning to who will help them to do their homework at night.

Moral Support and Encouragement

Parents also provide their children with other less tangible things like moral support and encouragement. Parents help to shape a child's perceptions about themselves and their self-identity. When a parent dies, the child loses one of the most important people in his or her life—someone who provides essential support and who is there during significant developmental milestones. This becomes a part of who a child is and who the child is becoming.

CHILD'S RELATIONSHIP WITH THE SURVIVING PARENT

When a parent dies, the child not only loses one parent, but also has a new and different mom or dad in the surviving parent. This is because the remaining parent is grieving as well. The surviving parent's grief affects every area of his or her life, as well as how the parent interacts with the child. To the child, this can be upsetting, and it can be a time of pain and confusion, both for the child and the parent. How the relationship between a child and parent is impacted after the death of one parent might vary based on many possible variables. The surviving parent and child (or children) must reestablish their relationship without the presence of the deceased parent (Christ, 2000). In Chapter 2, we discussed the various domains of family dynamics and how they are impacted after the death of a family member. It is also helpful to explore how to support healthy adaptation between the child and surviving parent following a death. This can be accomplished by a closer examination of the following Parent–Child Adaptive Tasks with which a parent and child might struggle when the other parent has died.

Parent–Child Adaptive Tasks

Reestablishing Security and Safety

After a parent dies, a child's sense of safety and security is compromised and the child often looks to the surviving parent for reassurance and support. This can be challenging for the surviving parent, who is also likely trying to find his or her own sense of security. Professionals providing support to families after the death of a parent can provide encouragement and offer opportunity for the surviving parent to explore ways he or she can reestablish a sense of security and safety with the child.

Children might have a myriad of worries and concerns after a parent dies. So it is helpful to identify the areas where children feel most vulnerable after the death of a parent. The following is a brief synopsis of things children might worry about after the death of a parent and how you can support the surviving parent to provide reassurance to the child.

Who Will Take Care of Me?

Children wonder and worry about what is going to happen to them after the death of a parent. They worry about who is going to take care of them and who is going to do all of the things for them that their parent who died did. When a parent dies, children lose one of the people who provides important interactions. Many times, they also (either temporarily or permanently) lose the attention of their surviving parent, as the surviving parent is grieving as well. These losses can affect the relationship with the surviving parent and other siblings and may also impact a child's sense of security.

What if My Other Parent Dies?

Some children worry about the safety of the surviving parent and are often concerned with this parent's health and well-being. Children might think, "If something bad has already happened to my mom, then it could happen to my dad." This brings about the worry and concern about who will take care of them if both parents die. As a result of this fear, some children might cling to the surviving parent, needing extra reassurance. Children also tend to stay close or cling to the surviving parent when they are missing the parent who died.

How to Help

Children who are experiencing this type of worry benefit from reassurance from their surviving parent. There are two major areas of concern that need to be addressed. First, encourage the parent to share with the child all the ways that the parent is taking care of himself or herself. Some examples of what the parent might say to the child are: "I am getting regular checkups with my doctor." "I am driving safely and being very careful." "I am eating healthy foods and taking care of myself physically." This type of reassurance will alleviate some of the child's worry.

Second, if the child is further concerned about what will happen to him or her if the surviving parent dies, too, there are steps that you can take with the surviving parent to provide additional reassurance. First, ask the surviving parent whether he or she has a plan for what happens to the child if the parent were to die. If there is no plan, remind the parent that it is important to establish a plan because the child is now aware that people can die. Further, it is impossible for the parent to completely reassure the child that nothing will happen to the parent. So, creating a plan and sharing that plan with the child is paramount.

Once you know that the parent has a plan, create an opportunity in the counseling setting or encourage the parent to set time aside at home with the child to discuss and share the plan. Questions the plan should answer are: Who will take care of me if you die? Where will I live? Will my brothers and sisters go with me? Where will I go to school? What will happen to my pets? What will happen to my things? Will I get to see my friends? Honestly answering these concerns can temper a child's worry over these important issues.

What if Someone Else in My Life Dies? What if I Die?

In addition to worrying about whether the surviving parent might die, thoughts about the death of others and their own death are common for children after someone in their life dies. It is important to provide an opportunity for children to express these concerns. This is often an ongoing conversation with their parents. Many adults find it difficult to discuss death and dying with their children. Rather, parents will often attempt to shelter their children from thinking about this topic. However, children fare better when they can share their concerns openly with the caring adults in their lives. In this way, children do not have to struggle with thoughts about death and dying on their own, but are able to process these difficult topics in a way that is safe and supportive (Figure 4.3).

Restoring Routines

As discussed in Chapter 2, most families operate within routines established, in part, by the pace of life, and by the daily choices of those in the family. Parents set daily schedules and routines, from sleeping habits and eating habits to shared family activities. Whether the home is extremely planned or more loosely defined, these routines provide a level of predictability to children. Predictability is an important part of creating a safe environment that supports healthy childhood development. The death of a parent can interrupt routines and compromise predictability. Though challenging, it is important for families to retain existing routines and, when needed, establish new routines within families.

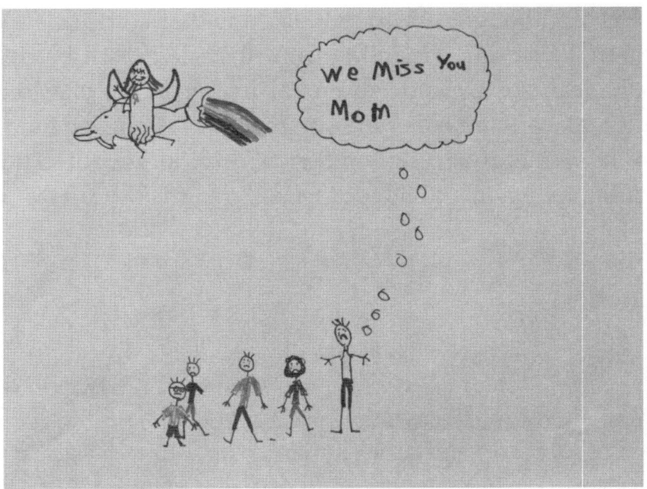

Figure 4.3 Artwork created by a preteen whose mom died.

How to Help

The importance of routines in the lives of children should be emphasized with the surviving parent. Engage the parent in a conversation about the routines prior to the death, how that changed (if at all) after the death, and what routines look like in the home now. This will help the parent identify where things have changed the most. Working with children, you can provide a space for the child to express how things have changed from the child's point of view since the death of the parent. This can help identify some of the routines that might have been compromised because of the death. It is also important to provide space in the counseling setting or encourage the parent at home to connect with the child on this topic and work together to reinstitute preexisting routines, or to establish new routines that meet the daily needs of the family.

Affirming and Maintaining Boundaries

Discipline is also an important part of establishing a safe environment for healthy psychological, social, and emotional development. Often boundaries, expectations of behavior, and consequences of misbehavior can be compromised after the death of a parent. It can be challenging for a surviving parent, who is grieving as well, to find the energy needed to hold children accountable to established rules and boundaries. It is also tempting to "soften the rules" temporarily because the children are grieving the death of someone in their lives. Although this is well-meaning and borne out of compassion for the children, removing discipline from their lives can be detrimental to their psychological, social, and emotional health. Also, children will often (unknowingly) take advantage of the situation and challenge long-established rules within the home. It is common for children to test these boundaries as they are learning to live in and adapt to a new reality.

How to Help

As professionals we should have resources available to parents with practical information and suggestions on establishing boundaries, discipline, and holding children accountable for their behavior in the home. There are a number of books and articles that address these issues that can be

(continued)

(*continued*)

provided as a reference to parents. The following are some basic tips you can share with parents specific to disciplining a bereaved child.

1. A child should be aware of clearly set boundaries and expectations of behavior in the home. Further, it should be emphasized to the child that the rules have not changed because of the death of one of the parents. Professionals can assist the parent with evaluating boundaries and expectations within the home, particularly if the parent is struggling with discipline since the death. Professionals can also provide the space in the counseling setting for parents and children to work together to reestablish clearly defined rules for the home.
2. If a child is acting out, the parent should first acknowledge that the child is grieving. Recognizing the reason a child might be acting out or testing boundaries is an important step for a surviving parent to take. Acknowledging a child's distress over the death of a parent is a step toward defusing the situation. For example, a parent might say to the child, "I see that you are having a very difficult time. I am wondering whether there is some way I might be of help to you." By taking this time, a parent is reinforcing important connections with the child and strengthening the foundation for a trusting, nurturing relationship. In other words, encourage parents to avoid going straight to instructing and correcting. First, the parent must acknowledge the child's grief and make himself or herself available to the child for help.
3. Grief should not be used as an excuse to misbehave. Though grief may be a reason the child is disobeying, it is detrimental to the child if grief is allowed to become an excuse. A grieving child must be held accountable for his or her behavior. Emphasize to the parent that this is how a child learns personal boundaries, how to interact with others, and other important social cues. Also, remind the parent to acknowledge the child's grief (see #2). Quite often by doing this, the situation is defused and there is no need for further intervention. If, however, the behavior persists, a parent might say to the child when he or she is misbehaving, "I know we are all having a difficult time since dad died, but hitting your sister is never okay." Then a parent might proceed with enforcing consequences for the behavior. By using this approach and this language, the parent is distinguishing between the child's grief and the behavior, while still holding the child accountable. In other words, *compassion and accountability can coexist.*

Adapting to New Roles and Responsibilities

Individuals within a family share a symbiotic relationship. Much like a healthy garden thrives from a balance of sun, water, good soil, and nurture, so, too, do families thrive from a balance of individual roles that are vital to routines, predictability, and security. When you remove one of the vital parts, families struggle corporately, and people within the family unit struggle individually to adapt their roles and responsibilities to accommodate the missing person. Sometimes this can cause difficulties within the family as individuals are challenged to evaluate their roles. For example, a surviving parent might struggle with taking on the role of both parents, or attempt to make up for the death of his or her spouse by taking on too much, risking becoming overextended. Children might also attempt to take on the role of the parent who died. Though not always the case, sometimes this is seen in older children of the same gender of the parent who died.

How to Help

Professionals can provide help to families to adapt to their new roles and responsibilities after the death of a parent. Here are some practical ideas for providing support and help.

1. Engage the surviving parent in discussion about what role the parent who died played in the family and in the life of the child. Help the parent identify the challenges that the death has brought to the family. What roles are missing? Are any of these roles vital?
2. Using child-friendly activities, ascertain from the child's perspective what roles the deceased parent played in the child's life and how the child has been impacted by the death.
3. Create a space in the counseling setting or encourage the parent at home to use activities to connect with the child on this topic. Encourage the parent to acknowledge the changes and how these changes have impacted the family. Encourage parents to identify practical solutions for the changing roles and how to fill the void.

Successful navigation of these four adaptive tasks is important and can be helpful to the family unit and to the individuals within the family. Professionals can provide the space, encouragement, and information the parent and the child need. As previously mentioned, families

(continued)

(*continued*)

come in many forms, so it is important for professionals to approach the surviving parent and the child as a learner, first and foremost. Then professionals can provide support, encouragement, and information in a trusting environment based on the parent's and child's expressed needs (Table 4.1).

Table 4.1 Parent–Child Adaptive Tasks After the Death of a Family Member

Parent–Child Adaptive Task	How to Help
Reestablishing security and safety	Identify what worries or fears a child might have about his or her own safety or the safety of others in the family. Provide opportunity for the parent and child to connect in the counseling setting. Work with the parent to create a plan for the child should the parent die. Encourage the parent to share this plan with the child. Provide space in the counseling setting for the child to express these concerns.
Restoring routines	Emphasize the importance of routines in the lives of a bereaved child and his or her parent. Use activities with the child (and parent) to express how things have changed since the death. Encourage the parent to connect with the child and to restore old routines and create new routines when old ones cannot be restored.
Affirming and maintaining boundaries	Have resources available for parents on the topic of boundaries, discipline, and holding children accountable for their behavior in the home. Practical information about how to clearly set boundaries will help a parent establish these needed guidelines.
Adapting to new roles and responsibilities	Provide space in the counseling setting for the parent to reflect on and discuss the challenges that the absence of the family member has brought to the family. What roles are missing?

SUMMARY

The death of a parent is a significant loss in a child's life and every area of life is impacted. Children depend on their parents to meet their daily needs. Not only do children adapt to the loss individually, but also as a family unit. The Parent–Child Adaptive Tasks provide a helpful framework for professionals to support families as they settle into a new normal after the death of a primary family member. Professionals can provide space in the support setting for parents to be supported in their own grief, as well as reflect on their role as parents, as they and their children adapt to the many changes brought about by the death.

REFERENCES

Christ, C. H. (2000). *Healing children's grief. Surviving a parent's death from cancer.* New York, NY: Oxford University Press.

Ellis, R. R., & Simmons, T. (2014). Coresident grandparents and their grandchildren: 2012. Retrieved from https://www.census.gov/content/dam/Census/library/publications/2014/demo/p20-576.pdf

Lofquist, D. (2011, September). Same-sex couple households. Retrieved from https://www.census.gov/prod/2011pubs/acsbr10-03.pdf

Silverman, P. R., & Worden, J. W. (1992). Children's reactions in the early months after the death of a parent. *American Journal of Orthopsychiatry, 62,* 93–104.

Vespa, J., Lewis, J. M., & Kreider, R. M. (2013, August). America's families and living arrangements: 2012. Retrieved from https://www.census.gov/prod/2013pubs/p20-570.pdf

Death of Other Family Members

When one person is missing the whole world seems empty.
—*Pat Schweibert*, Tear Soup: A Recipe for Healing After Loss

In this chapter we take a closer look at how the death of various family members impacts a child's life. Not only are children affected by the death of a parent or primary caregiver, they are also affected by the death of other members of their family. Many of the same considerations after the death of a parent might also apply to the death of other family members. A child's reactions to death in the family are influenced by many factors. Some of these include the closeness of the relationship, whether the person who died was a part of the dynamics of the family, and the presence of this person in the child's everyday life. In the case of a sibling or extended family member living in the same household with the child, it is likely that many of the Parent–Child Adaptive Tasks discussed in Chapter 4 will apply to adaptation after the death in these circumstances. Professionals should be prepared to discuss the impact of the death of other family members within this context, just as we would in the case of the death of a parent.

There are also special circumstances related to the death of other family members that are unique to these types of losses in a child's life. For example, the relationship siblings have with one another differs greatly from the relationship they have with their parents. This is also true of the relationship children have with their grandparents, favorite aunt or uncle, or cousins. Keep in mind, however, that the *Universal Realities of Grief* discussed in Chapter 1 apply to any death impacting a child's life; namely, that grief is best understood through the perspective of the person experiencing the death. As professionals, we should position ourselves as learners. We should seek to understand a family's culture, beliefs, traditions, and dynamics in order to provide a safe space for a child and the family to cope with their grief. We lay a groundwork in more general terms regarding relationships children have with both immediate and extended family that can be applied to a number of family circumstances.

THE DEATH OF A SIBLING

Like the death of a parent, the death of a sibling can also be a life-altering experience for a child. Sibling relationships inform a child's understanding of how the world works and provide a context in which personality, preferences, social norms, and interactions with others are developed. The death of a sibling not only impacts a child's daily life, it also impacts the child's understanding of his or her sense of self and future. In addition, children feel the impact of a brother or sister's death on their entire family and worry that their family is forever changed (Hogan, 2008). In this section, we discuss the strength of the sibling relationship, specific factors that impact that relationship, and how it influences a child's grief after the death of a sibling. It is important to note, however, that there are a variety of types of relationships that siblings have with one another and that the information provided here are generalizations. There is no replacement for listening to a child express what his or her relationship with the sibling meant to the child and how it is impacting daily life.

The Strength of the Sibling Relationship

Sibling relationships are often unique and irreplaceable. Many siblings grow up in the same household and share a similar history and experience. They often create bonds that are strong and lasting. In some families, siblings are each other's allies, protectors, and mentors, as well as each other's playmates, rivals, and role models (Davies, 1995). Often, siblings learn important life lessons from one another and are each other's first friend or real relationship outside of their parents. Siblings might know each other better than their parents know them, as they share many secrets and tend to confide in one another. They often teach each other how to play, negotiate, work through a fight, laugh, and interact with others in social settings. Siblings also might imagine a full life together. Sometimes these relationships are mostly loving though competitive; other times sibling relationships can be contentious or even nonexistent though they share a home with one another. In this way, sibling relationships can be complicated.

Not only can sibling relationships be complex, but they can also change over time. Some siblings are quite compatible, whereas others argue and don't get along. Many sibling relationships are a combination of both compatibility and strife (Davies, 1995). Either way, the sibling relationship has a strong influence on the way a child understands and interacts with the world. For these reasons, the death of a sibling can have a profound impact on both a child's outlook, and on the child's daily life. How the child is impacted depends greatly on a number of factors. It is helpful to explore the sibling relationship in the context of three spheres—sibling companionship, sibling rivalry, and sibling reciprocity.

Sibling Companionship

Siblings share many life experiences together as companions within the context of their family. As with anyone sharing the same space, sometimes they get along with one another and other times they might fuss and fight. In this regard, they are sojourners who share a family, a culture, and many life experiences. They learn about life together, sharing many experiences of new discovery. They keep each other's secrets and are often "partners in crime." Siblings develop friendships, many of which last throughout their lives. They learn about and interpret life together as they experience the world and the many challenges of childhood. Although some siblings might be closer than others, they still share a history together and they become who they are as a result of their relationship with one another. We go into more detail about this in the section: "Other Factors That Impact Sibling Relationships."

Sibling Rivalry

The rivalry between siblings is often an important part of how children carve out their own unique self-identities within the context of their family, friends, and community settings. Siblings will often compete with one another, whether consciously or unconsciously. Some of the things they compete for are their parents' and other family members' attention, to have things their way, to have their own possessions, and to have their voice heard. As they compete for this attention, they are formulating their own unique roles within the family context. In the process, some siblings might develop a more contentious relationship with one another, rather than a friendship. This can sometimes manifest itself in strong opposition to one another. These dynamics are important for professionals to understand, as they can influence a child's grief after the death of a sibling.

Sibling Reciprocity

Younger siblings in a family will often identify with one or more of their older siblings. At times when a child identifies with a sibling, he or she strives to emulate qualities, styles, or personality characteristics of that sibling.

For example, the child might want to dress like, tag along with, or behave like one of the older siblings. Older siblings might see themselves as the protectors, or feel a sense of responsibility for the younger sibling. This is sometimes reinforced by older siblings "babysitting" their younger sibling, or taking on other roles of parenting (e.g., changing diapers, feeding, tucking into bed).

Further, interplay among siblings provides a setting where siblings influence the development of one another. For example, siblings might share a similar sense of humor or shared interest in certain activities. This exchange between siblings reinforces particular characteristics and behaviors that mark shared experiences of childhood and life. In other words, siblings can take on characteristics that are similar to their brothers and sisters.

Other Factors That Impact Sibling Relationships

The sibling relationship is influenced by a number of factors. These include birth order, gender, age, and personality of each child within the family. For example, a child's place in the birth order of the family will have an impact on the child's personality and relationship with other siblings. If the oldest sibling dies, the middle child now becomes the oldest child in the family. Or, if the youngest dies, the middle child becomes the youngest. Children within a family might struggle with these changes as they adapt to new roles or ways of relating to others in the family.

Family size, dynamics, and circumstances also impact the sibling relationship. Children in large families (four or more children) often have a different level of responsibility than children in smaller families (three or fewer children). Also, there is typically a wider range of ages in larger families with children in different developmental stages of life, which impacts sibling relationships. As mentioned in Chapter 2, the various domains of family dynamics will also impact sibling interactions with one another.

Other important considerations are the circumstances of the family and how these circumstances impact the sibling relationships. For example, in blended families sibling roles and dynamics shift as step-siblings adapt to the new family dynamics. Some step-sibling relationships might be contentious, whereas others might provide the opportunity for new experiences and perspectives. In divorced or fractured families, siblings might live together or they might live separately. They also might take opposing sides if the separation was particularly difficult. They can also become more reliant on each other depending on the attention and involvement of their parents in their lives after the separation.

Understanding sibling relationships and the factors that influence them are an important part of a child's story, both before and after the death of a sibling.

The relationship a child had with the deceased sibling will have a direct impact on the child's grief. It is important for professionals to have an understanding of what the relationship was like with that sibling in order to better understand the individual needs of that particular child.

Impact of the Death of a Sibling and How to Help Children

Parent–Child Relationship

As discussed previously in Chapter 4, the relationship a child has with his or her caregiver is one of the top factors impacting a child's health after a death, including the death of a sibling. This relationship can sometimes be strained after the death of a sibling because a child's parents are also grieving the death of a child. Grieving the death of a child is particularly difficult for parents and brings with it challenges particular to this type of loss. Bereaved parents often express guilt that they could not keep their child from dying. In addition, they fear that they cannot continue to live with or accept their child's death. They also express anger over why it had to be their child. In our work with bereaved parents, many have often said, "This should not have happened. I am supposed to die before my child. A parent should never have to bury a child."

Both grief and parenting take a huge amount of mental, physical, and emotional energy. Because of this, it can be quite challenging for a bereaved parent to provide the same level of time and attention to parenting. Children are often acutely aware that their parents are suffering and over time come to realize that the death of their sibling changes their parents (Hogan, 2008). Most children are sensitive to their parents' pain, sadness, and sense of loss (Jonas-Simpson, Steele, Granek, Davies, & O'Leary, 2015). Professionals can use the Parent–Child Adaptive Tasks as outlined in Chapter 4 (see Table 4.1) when counseling and supporting children and their families after the death of a sibling. Helping parents and children restore balance in the home is a top priority because the parent–child relationship is the top influential factor in the health of children.

After the death of a sibling, children's sense of security can be compromised as they now are aware that death is a possibility for themselves and those around them. Routines can be interrupted as everyone in the home is grieving and energy levels are low. For this same reason, disciplining surviving children can also be a challenge. Quite often, established boundaries are crossed without consequence. And finally, members of the family are shifting and moving as they adapt to new roles in response to the absence of one of their own.

Professionals should avoid judgement and be patient with bereaved parents as they are grieving the death of their child and, at the same time, trying to continue to provide for the needs of their surviving children. However, professionals should also seek to empower bereaved parents. This can be accomplished by providing parents with support, encouragement, and resources about parenting bereaved children and how to help their children after the death of a sibling.

Sense of Self

Children's *sense of self* can be defined as their perception of who they are and who they believe themselves to be. A child's sense of self manifests itself in the different settings in which he or she lives. These settings might include family, school, or neighborhood, to name a few. Depending on the relationship a child had with the sibling who died, he or she might struggle with the sense of self in the context of this relationship. For example, a child whose only sibling dies might struggle with the thought that he or she is now an only child. Or a middle child might have a difficult time adjusting to being the oldest child in the household after the death of an older sibling.

In light of their loss, children can also redefine their sense of self. For example, when Chad was 12, his older brother was killed in a car accident. When meeting with his school counselor, Chad reflected, "Before my brother died, I thought I could do anything. But, since his death, I feel like I can't do anything right." The death of Chad's brother directly impacted Chad's confidence and self-image. At the same time, children's confidence might increase after the death of a sibling because they realize they are stronger than they thought they were. After the death of her older brother, Sally reflected, "I have learned things about myself that I never knew when my brother was alive. I have gone through a lot since his death. It has brought me out of my shell and I am doing things now that I never thought I could do." When working with children, professionals might see many variations of these two examples.

Preexisting Relationship With the Deceased Sibling

As discussed previously in "The Strength of the Sibling Relationship" section in this chapter, the sibling relationship is a central factor in a child's growth and development. In the same way, a child's grief is impacted by the preexisting relationship with the deceased sibling. For example, Amy was 6 when her 9-year-old sister, Emily, died unexpectedly. Amy looked up to Emily and they were constant playmates. Because of their close relationship, Amy not only lost a sister, but also lost her best friend and companion. This is a common experience for children who had a positive relationship with the sibling who died.

Conversely, Jake was only 18 months older than his brother Scott. Though they were close, they were very competitive and argued with each other often. The day before Scott was killed in an all-terrain vehicle accident, the two brothers got into a heated argument and Jake told his brother that he "hated him and didn't want anything to do with him." After Scott's death, Jake became very angry any time someone brought up Scott. He became argumentative with his parents and began isolating himself from his and Scott's mutual friends. Jake's teacher recommended he talk to his school counselor. After several sessions with his counselor, Jake disclosed that he was feeling very guilty about his last conversation with his brother. It is not unusual when there was a contentious relationship with the person who died for a sibling to experience intense feelings of guilt, anger, or regret.

Loss of Innocence

The death of a sibling impacts a child's sense of innocence in a variety of ways. After the death of a sibling, a child becomes keenly aware of the stark reality that people their age can die. They now know something about life (and death) that their friends do not know. This loss of innocence might cause children to feel different from their friends. Depending on the type of death, a child might also be faced with thinking about circumstances related to the death that are far beyond their age or level of maturity. For example, after 15-year-old Elijah's older sister died, Elijah began to worry about how his family was going to cope. He felt like he should be able to fill his sister's shoes, especially because his single mother really depended on his sister to help care for the younger siblings in the family (Figure 5.1).

Loss of a Future With the Sibling

Children grieving the death of a sibling experience sadness that their deceased sibling no longer gets to enjoy life with them. This includes both big and small activities. For example, a child might express sadness that his or her deceased sibling does not get to enjoy fun family times or meals together. Children not only lose a playmate or confidant in the present, but they also lose someone who potentially would have been a lifelong friend or companion (Davies, 1999). In the same way, they might reflect on their sibling's absence at milestone events like getting a driver's license, graduation, or their first kiss. This can also create an added challenge with milestones, such as birthdays, as the child continues to grow. For example, younger siblings might have a difficult time when they turn the age that their older sibling was when he or she died. It is helpful when children are encouraged to continue the connection with

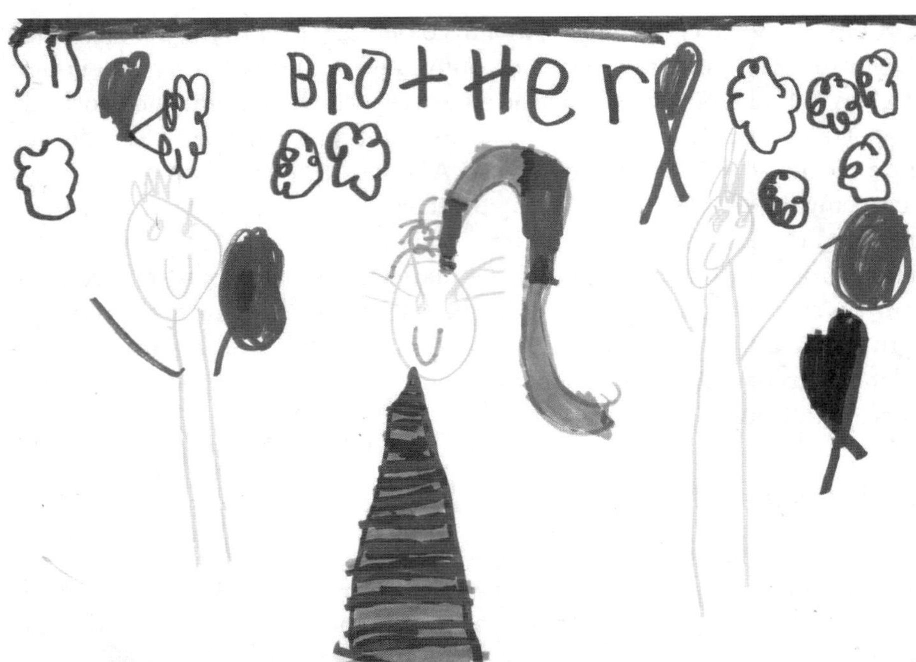

Figure 5.1 Artwork created by a younger child whose brother died.

their deceased sibling as they grow older (Packman, Horsley, Davies, & Kramer, 2006). This is further discussed in the Encouraging Continuing Bonds section in Chapter 7.

Guilt

A child might experience a sense of guilt after the death of a sibling. The child might struggle with accepting that he or she gets to keep growing up, experiencing life, and being with family and friends, while the sibling is missing out on all of these things. Quite simply, sometimes children feel guilty because they are alive and their siblings are not (Hogan, 2008). It is common for a child to express, "I don't feel right about laughing and having fun when my sister is dead." It is also common for children to feel guilt over something they did or said before their sibling died. They might even believe that they caused the death in some way. For example, children might think that had they been nicer to their sibling, their sibling would not have died.

It is important for professionals to be patient with a child experiencing guilt after a sibling's death. Attempting to rationalize with a child about the death in order to "take away" or "fix" a child's guilt should be avoided. Processing their sense of guilt is an integral part of children's struggle to adapt to their new reality. Professionals should provide a setting where children can express their thoughts and feelings, whatever those feelings might be. We discuss this further in Chapter 8, in the section, "Creating a Safe Space for Support."

Family Adaptation After the Death of a Sibling

Each person in a family unit is a part of the whole. When one part is missing, everything shifts as members adapt to accommodate for the absence of the deceased person. Just as when a parent dies, families adapt and change after the death of a sibling. These changes are influenced by a number of factors. One factor is the health of the parents and their reaction to the death. Another factor is the relationship between the parents and their children. Additionally, the preexisting relationship of the child to a deceased sibling influences family adaptation. The varying grief reactions of the children in the family are also influenced. In order to assist families as they adapt to the death of one of their members, professionals should refer to the domains of family dynamics in Chapter 2 and apply these concepts to the death of a sibling.

DEATH OF A GRANDPARENT

For many children, their first experience with the death of someone in their family is the death of a grandparent (Corr & Corr, 1996). How a child reacts to the death of a grandparent might vary based on a number of circumstances. These might include how bonded they are to that grandparent, whether that grandparent lived in the same home with the child, or how often the child saw that grandparent. In this section, we look at the strength of the grandparent–grandchild relationship and the different circumstances that might impact a child's grief after the death of a grandparent.

The Strength of the Grandparent–Grandchild Relationship

Grandparents have a unique relationship with their grandchildren that is often quite different than the relationship they have with their own children. For one, they are not the primary caregiver for their grandchild (see the section

"Grandparents Raising Grandchildren" for considerations when they are). Because they are not the primary caregiver, they are able to focus on other aspects of the relationship like fun activities and teachable moments.

Grandparents also provide their grandchildren with a connection to their family's history. They are often the ones who pass down stories that their grandparents shared with them about fun times, hard times, and overcoming the challenges of life. In this way, they are the keepers of the family history. They are also the bearers of many family heirlooms, often passing these down to their children and grandchildren as they get older. Many grandparents live close to their grandchildren and serve as babysitters when parents need a night out. They are teachers to their grandchildren sharing with them reflections about life, the world, and how certain things work.

It is common for adults and professionals to assume that a child will not grieve as intently over the death of a grandparent as this is the "natural" order of things. Professionals should avoid this assumption. When children are very close to their grandparents and have a strong bond with them, they will typically be profoundly impacted by the death (Crenshaw, 1990). Rather, professionals should provide a context for children to remember and share their thoughts and feelings. Following are a few circumstances that might impact a child's grief after the death of a grandparent. As a reminder, these are generalizations and do not apply in every situation.

Circumstances That Impact a Child's Grief Over the Death of a Grandparent

Grandparents Living Nearby or in the Home With Their Grandchildren

Grandparents who live nearby or even in the same home with their grandchildren are more likely to form a close bond. They are also likely to play a significant role in daily routines and family dynamics. Because of this, a child's grief after the grandparent's death might be more intense than if the grandparent lived at a great distance and the child saw him or her only occasionally. In some cases grief over the death of a grandparent can be as intense as grief over the death of a parent or sibling because the child interacted with the grandparent on a daily basis.

Grandparents With Life Limiting or Terminal Illnesses

Another circumstance that impacts a child's grief after the death of a grandparent is when a grandparent has a life-limiting or terminal illness. One of the factors that might impact a child's grief in this type of circumstance is the amount of contact the child had with the ill grandparent. In some families, aging or ill grandparents might have a room in the home and everyone in the family pitches in with their care. In other families, children might be shielded from the realities of the illness. Whatever the circumstance, a child is impacted by the long-term or terminal illness of a grandparent. Wediscuss anticipated death reactions in Chapter 3 and provide ideas for helping a child cope with the illness.

Grandparents Raising Grandchildren

Grandparents raising their grandchildren is a growing phenomenon in our society (Ellis & Simmons, 2014). When a grandparent takes on the responsibility of raising a grandchild, this creates a completely different dynamic in the grandparent–grandchild relationship. In this situation, the grandparent is acting as the child's parent. He or she ceases to be the grandparent and must take on the role of a parent. Information provided in Chapter 4 about the death of a parent will apply in this circumstance.

Parents Grieving the Death of Their Parents

How a parent grieves the death of his or her own parent has a great impact on the grief of a grandchild. As previously mentioned, grief takes a large amount of energy and can impact a parent's ability to provide consistency and to maintain normal routines within the home. The duration and intensity of the parent's grief can permanently alter the home environment. This might be the first time some children have ever seen their parent cry (Corr & Corr, 1996). It is not unusual for parents to bring their children to counseling after the death of a grandparent out of the parent's own need for grief support. Parents will not always acknowledge this, or might not even be aware of it. Professionals should offer resources to parents about self-care in the midst of grief, in addition to providing opportunities for children to explore, express, and find support for their grief over the death of their grandparent.

DEATH OF OTHER FAMILY MEMBERS

As discussed previously, the death of someone in a child's life is both a personal and corporate experience. Information provided about how grief impacts a child's life in the first few chapters of this book can be applied when the death is a family member other than the parent, sibling, or grandparent. Whoever it is who has died in a child's life, professionals should seek to understand how each individual child is grieving and the surrounding circumstances of that child's particular situation. Some of these include the dynamics within the family, what the child's relationship with the deceased person was like, and how the child's grief is manifesting itself. Whether or not a person was a part of a child's everyday life, a child might still grieve that person's death. At the least, the death of a family member brings thoughts of death and dying to the forefront of a child's mind. Professionals should seek to understand how a death has impacted a child's life. They should provide support and resources to children and their families regardless of which member of the family has died (Figures 5.2 and 5.3).

My Brother

I will never forget his smile,

I will never forget his eyes,

I will never forget his laugh,

I will never forget his heart,

I will never forget his ideas,

I will never forget the way he cared,

I will never forget how active he was,

I will never forget the way his voice sounded,

I will never forget the dreams he told me,

I will never forget the way he loved me,

I will never forget him!

Figure 5.2 Poem created by a preteen whose brother died.

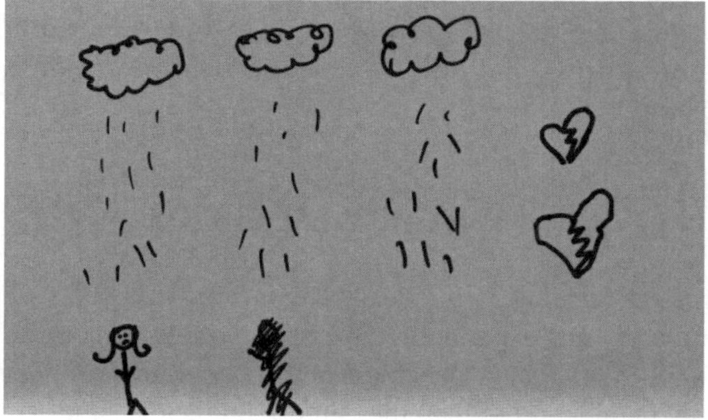

Figure 5.3 Artwork created by a younger child whose grandma died.

SUMMARY

Children have many meaningful relationships in their lives. It is important that we allow children to define what these relationships mean to them and how the death of a person in their life has impacted them. The sibling relationship may involve important shared bonds that will impact grief when a sibling dies. Grandparents provide children with a unique relationship, as they bring with them important connections to family history and culture. Whatever the relationship might be, when children experience the death of someone in their lives, they need care, compassion, and patience as they incorporate that loss into their present reality.

REFERENCES

Corr, C. A., & Corr, D. M. (Eds.). (1996). *Handbook of childhood death and bereavement.* New York, NY: Springer Publishing.

Crenshaw, D. A. (1990). *Bereavement: Counseling the grieving through the life cycle.* New York, NY: Continuum.

Davies, B. (1995). Toward siblings' understanding and perspective of death. In E. A. Grollman (Ed.), *Bereaved children and teens: A support guide for parents and professionals* (pp. 61–74). Boston, MA: Beacon Press.

Davies, B. (1999). *Shadows in the sun: The experiences of sibling bereavement in childhood.* New York, NY: Routledge.

Ellis, R. R., & Simmons, T. (2014). Coresident grandparents and their grandchildren: 2012. Retrieved from https://www.census.gov/content/dam/Census/library/publications/2014/demo/p20-576.pdf

Hogan, N. (2008). Sibling loss: Issues for children and adolescents. In K. Doka & A. Tucci (Eds.), *Living with grief: Children and adolescents* (pp. 159–174). Washington, DC: Hospice Foundation of America.

Jonas-Simpson, C., Steele, R., Granek, L., Davies, B., & O'Leary, J. (2015). Always with me: Understanding experiences of bereaved children whose baby sibling died. *Death Studies, 39,* 242–251.

Packman, W., Horsley, H., Davies, B., & Kramer, R. (2006). Sibling bereavement and continuing bonds. *Death Studies, 30,* 817–841.

CHAPTER 6

Factors That Promote Health in Grieving Children

Health is a state of complete physical, mental and social well-being, and not merely the absence of disease or infirmity.

—World Health Organization*

There are many protective and promotive factors that support the health of bereaved children. Many of these factors are inherent in a child's personal attributes, his or her social and environmental surroundings, home life, and culture. Some of these factors include having the support of family and friends and maintaining continuing bonds with the person who died. Another helpful factor includes being around other children who have also experienced the death of someone close. This chapter provides professionals with information about these elements and their importance in the lives of children.

A POSITIVE PARENT–CHILD RELATIONSHIP

The foundation of a positive parent–child relationship is loving, warm, and consistent interaction between a parent and child. These underpinnings provide the setting for a relationship between a parent and child that promotes resilience, a positive self-image, confidence, a hopeful outlook, and the basis for positive social relationships (Haine, Ayers, Sandler, & Wolchik, 2008).

Fundamentals of a Positive Parent–Child Relationship

Childhood bereavement research and practice identify the relationship a bereaved child has with his or her parent (or primary caregiver) as a top

*Reprinted from World Health Organization. Constitution of WHO: principles, Copyright 1946. URL: http://www.who.int/about/mission/en/

indicator of a child's health after the death of someone in the child's life (Haine, Wolchik, Sandler, Millsap, & Ayers, 2006; Worden, 1996). Because of this, we have provided much information throughout this text for professionals regarding the parent–child relationship, and tips for supporting and encouraging positive adaptation after a death. In addition, professionals should have a working knowledge of the fundamentals of a positive parent and child relationship. Through our work with bereaved children and their parents, we have identified a number of fundamentals that denote a positive relationship between a parent and child.

Open, Accepting, and Nonjudgmental Communication

The way a parent communicates with his or her child is an important component that supports a positive parent–child relationship. Professionals should encourage parents to communicate with their children in an open, accepting, and nonjudgmental way. Having this type of communication provides a context for bereaved children to feel comfortable approaching their parent (Silverman, Weiner, & Elad, 1995). Children might have a number of questions, concerns, thoughts, or ideas that they want to share with their parent. An open relationship between a parent and child helps a child feel comfortable approaching the parent with questions.

One way professionals can encourage parents to establish this positive communication with their child is by promoting an interactive conversational style. Quite often, parents communicate with their children through a series of probing questions as opposed to a conversation style that actively engages their child. Interactive conversation includes storytelling, reminiscing, processing ideas, and telling jokes, to name a few. When parents are able to have back and forth conversations by sharing stories, funny memories, or serious thoughts, children often reciprocate with stories of their own. For example, a mother might share a story about something that happened to her when she was a child or about her everyday life. This type of communication encourages mutual understanding between a child and parent as they learn about one another. It also provides a context for a child to identify with the parent as they swap stories about life.

When children are comfortable expressing their thoughts and feelings openly with their parents, they are able to better relate to their parents. Further, when parents are approachable, bereaved children are able to disclose their thoughts and feelings about the person who died, while also feeling accepted and understood by their parent (Hurd, 1999). This is an important part of a child's ability to process the death, what the death of this person means to the child now, and how to incorporate it into the present reality.

Mutual Trust

Mutual trust is another important component of a positive parent–child relationship. This component is reinforced by open communication between a parent and child as discussed in the preceding section. A child who is able to openly share, emote, and engage with the parent and receive acknowledgment in return, is able to establish a mutually trusting relationship with that parent.

Honesty also promotes mutual trust in the parent–child relationship. As referenced earlier in the book, professionals should encourage parents to share age-appropriate, factual information with their children about the death. This might include how a person died and the circumstances surrounding the death. This will reinforce children's belief that they can trust their parent to tell them the truth. Telling children the truth about a death as a result of suicide, for example, will help children begin processing the details of the death with care-givers present. Not telling children the truth, or the details of the death, can be very confusing, especially if they overhear details from other family members.

Another element of building trust is for parents to consistently do what they say they are going to do. Predictability and follow through are as important to building trust as openness and honesty. When a parent is consistent and follows through with his or her commitments to the child, the parent strengthens the bond of trust he or she has with the child. All of these things reinforce a child's sense that the parent cares about the child and the experience that the child is going through. As professionals we can encourage parents to be open, honest, and consistent with their children (Figure 6.1).

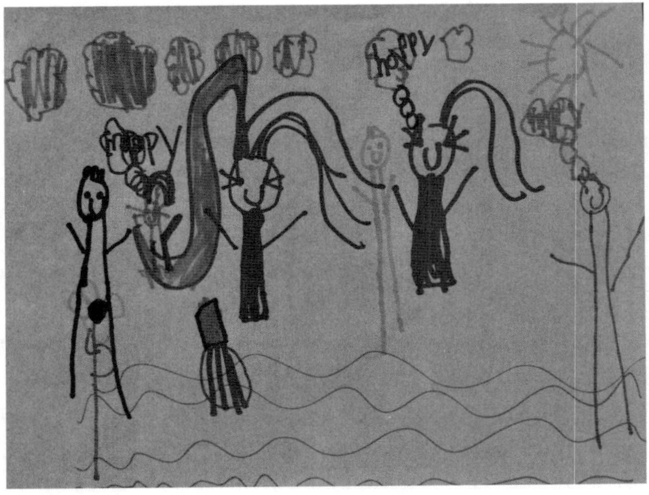

Figure 6.1 Artwork created by a young child whose brother died.

Nurturing Interactions

First and foremost, nurturing is how parents demonstrate care and concern for the well-being of their children. Professionals should seek to understand how parents nurture their children, and should help parents identify practical ways to interact with their children in nurturing ways. For example, parents nurture their children when they validate how their children are feeling. They validate their children's feelings by acknowledging what is bothering their children and by listening to them express their thoughts and feelings about their experiences and, in turn, normalizing their children's experiences (Grollman, 1990).

After Fred's dad's death, one night at bedtime, he said to his mom, "I really miss Dad and sometimes at night I feel very sad," to which his mom replied, "I get sad because I miss Dad, too. It is okay for us to feel this way." They shared a hug and then went on with their normal bedtime routine. Encouraging parents to spend quality time like this with their children and to acknowledge their children's feelings provides the context for parents to offer guidance, understanding, and support as children adapt to their loss.

Children are also nurtured when they feel a sense of friendship and companionship with their parents. Although parents have to be disciplinarians, role models, and heads of the household, it is also important that parents establish a friendship with their children. For example, professionals should encourage parents to spend time with their children playing games, playing make believe, coloring, drawing, and other types of fun activities that make children feel safe. Friendly interactions between children and their parents reinforce to children that their parents are glad they are in the world and that they are not alone in their grief.

Knowing and Respecting Their Child's Personality and Preferences

Another essential component of a positive parent–child relationship is a parent knowing the child. Each child has his or her own unique personality and preferences for how the child feels most comfortable being in the world. Professionals can encourage parents and give them ideas about how they can interact with their children at home to get to know them better. It is important for parents to understand that their children are growing and changing. This will impact their likes, dislikes, and individual preferences. Using some of the other components provided in this section, parents can get to know their children better. Professionals should be patient with parents, however, as they are quite possibly grieving as well and it takes much energy to spend quality time with their children.

Table 6.1 Fundamentals of a Positive Parent–Child Relationship	
Open, accepting, and nonjudgmental communication	Communication that fosters warm feelings between bereaved children and their parents
Mutual trust	The ability for children to openly share, emote, and engage their parents and receive acknowledgment in return
Nurturing interactions	Interactions that reinforce to children that their parents are glad they are in the world and that they are not alone in their grief
Knowing and respecting their child's personality and preferences	Recognition that each child has his or her own unique personality and preferences for how the child feels most comfortable being in the world
Appropriate, predictable, and consistent discipline	Discipline that does not degrade or harm a child, but is planned, structured, and implemented with purpose by a parent

Appropriate, Predictable, and Consistent Discipline

Appropriate, predictable, and consistent discipline is an important factor that promotes a positive parent–child relationship. Appropriate discipline is not reactive, but rather is planned, structured, and purposefully implemented by a parent. It also never degrades a child, nor physically, mentally, or emotionally harms a child. In the case of a bereaved child, parents should first consider how grief is impacting the child before enacting punishment for misbehavior, as quite often a bereaved child will act out because of grief. It is important that a parent acknowledges a child's grief and normalizes that experience, even when discipline is necessary. For specific information to share with your clients regarding discipline, refer to the "Affirming and Maintaining Boundaries" section in Chapter 4 (Table 6.1).

EXPRESSION AND VALIDATION OF GRIEF

Another factor that promotes health in bereaved children is the ability for children to express their grief and to have their experience validated. Bereaved children and their parents often lack a context for understanding whether what they are experiencing is "normal" under the circumstances. Often, parents worry that they might be missing something or that their children might need more professional help. Children often feel as if they are the only people dealing with the death of someone close to them. They will express that they do not know anyone else among their friends who has experienced their specific type of loss.

Professionals can provide support to children and their families by creating space in the support setting for children and their parents to express their grief in the way that feels most natural to them, and by offering the space for their grief to be normalized and supported. As professionals we can create a space where children and families under our care *feel felt*, or put another way, feel like someone "gets" them (Schuurman & DeCristofaro, 2007). For example, support groups provide an opportunity for children and their parents to express themselves and be with others going through a similar situation. Grief-support groups help to normalize a family's grief and validate that they are not the only people going through the loss of someone they love (Figure 6.2).

Children express their grief in a variety of ways. Children might want to talk about the person who died and they might also want to share their grief with others. It is important to note, however, that grief is expressed in more ways than just talking. Some children prefer to express their grief through activities such as writing a letter to the person who died, drawing a picture of a favorite memory of the person who died, or painting a picture of what their grief looks like.

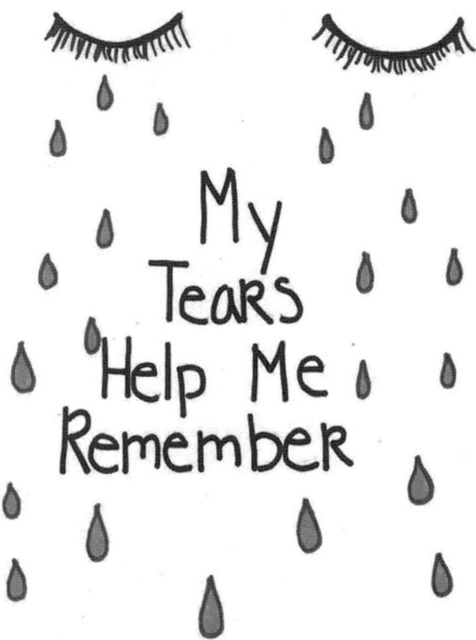

Figure 6.2 Artwork created by a teenager whose mom died.

Children may also express their grief through play. Play is a language that children often use to express their thoughts and feelings. Play provides the opportunity to release big emotions that often produce big energy. Play also gives children the chance to reenact key aspects of their loss. For example, children might reenact a car crash with toy cars in an attempt to make sense of what happened if their dad died in a car crash. Similarly, given the proper funeral-related toys and figurines, children will often reenact what the funeral looked and felt like to them.

Another way they might express their grief is through memorializing activities. Children will do things in honor of their deceased loved one. They might save items they find around the house that remind them of the person and keep them in a special place. Many children cherish pictures of the person who died that remind them of a favorite memory or time with that person. Other ideas for memorializing are for children to celebrate a person's birthday, visit the cemetery, or create things in the person's memory (Figure 6.3).

Providing opportunities for children to convey their thoughts and feelings about the loss, as mentioned, is important for the ventilation of feelings. Also important is that these thoughts and feelings are supported when expressed. At times, adults might be uncomfortable with certain reactions they may see in children. They might, as a result, verbally attempt to redirect or make things okay by saying, "It's okay; you don't have to feel sad because your dad is in a better place," or similar statements. Though well intended, this type of reaction to a child's expression of grief misses the opportunity to normalize and validate what the child is experiencing. Professionals should provide information

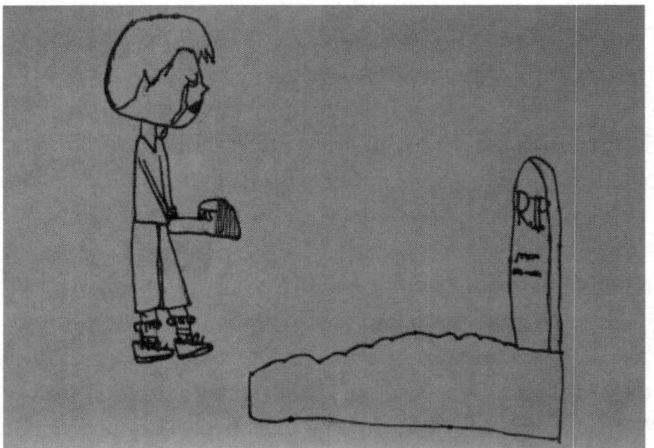

Figure 6.3 Artwork created by an older child whose dad died.

to adults supporting bereaved children about the types of reactions they might see in children, as well as helpful resources that are available in their community.

Children fare better when their grief experience is normalized. When children are able to meet with other children going through a similar situation, they realize that they are not alone and that what they are experiencing is normal. When the adults in their lives acknowledge and validate their experiences, children often feel more comfortable expressing their grief and they also feel as though someone understands what they are going through.

A CHILD'S SENSE OF CONTROL

An important factor that promotes health in children is the ability for bereaved children to be able to regain and retain a sense of control (Sandler, Wolchik, & Ayers, 2007). After someone dies, children often lose a sense of control over their lives. Because of the death, they might feel that the world is no longer a safe, predictable place. In the years after a death, it is imperative for children to reestablish a sense of control. It is important to provide options and allow children to exercise control within the counseling setting as this can reestablish a sense of control to their lives. Reestablishing a sense of control involves being able to make choices and having those choices matter.

Children should be provided opportunities to retain control in a variety of settings. This includes at home, school, or any number of environments. This also includes being allowed to create solutions so that they may solve their own problems. In a grief-support setting, children are typically offered many ways to regain control. Some examples of this include having an option of activities to choose from, having the option to "pass," and deciding whether to talk or not to talk within the group setting.

Another way to help children with their sense of control is letting them participate in activities that allow them to interject their own ideas. In addition, ideas for how children can react to their situation or to other people should be given, as well as ideas for how to cope, which are included at the end of this chapter.

Bereaved children are also able to regain a sense of control by being empowered by the adults around them. Adults in children's lives should help to provide the tools children need to be in control of their own choices. Another practical way to regain a sense of control after a death is to allow children to help plan and participate in the funeral. Children can also participate in the establishment of a new normal in the family. This could include creating new family traditions or new family rituals.

POSITIVE SELF-ESTEEM

Positive self-esteem is an important factor in contributing to the health of bereaved children (Greeff & Berquin, 2004). After the death of someone in their lives, children face a number of challenges. These include going back to school and dealing with questions and comments from their peers to adapting to the changing environment at home. Challenges such as these can be taxing on the way children view themselves. How children navigate these difficulties can have a direct impact on their self-esteem.

Professionals can provide a space in the support setting for children to explore and work through these challenges. They can work with children to set small achievable goals, providing the opportunity for small successes that bolster children's self-esteem. The can also help children problem solve some of the challenging situations they have or will encounter. This helps children establish a plan and heightens the likelihood of a positive outcome, strengthening children's sense of positive self-regard. Professionals can encourage children after some of these small accomplishments.

Professionals can provide parents with resources about how to support and strengthen their child's self-esteem. As previously mentioned, parents have a unique opportunity to positively impact their child's health after the death of someone close to them. Receiving acknowledgment, encouragement, and support from a parent can serve as an anchor for the child as he or she navigates the many challenges and new changes brought about by the loss.

HEALTHY COPING SKILLS

People develop coping skills as they experience the ebbs and flows of life. These skills are developed over time throughout a person's life. After the death of someone in a child's life, he or she will apply many of these ways of coping to the challenges and changes brought about by the death. In fact, many behaviors are an attempt to cope, often unbeknownst to the bereaved child. Further, coping with grief can be understood as the way a bereaved child handles, manages, and navigates grief after a loss. Some ways of coping are healthier than others. Sometimes children might cope with grief in ways that are harmful, bringing added challenges to an already difficult situation.

Professionals can support bereaved children by providing space for them to identify ways they are coping with their grief that are both healthy and unhealthy, and explore ideas for improving coping when existing patterns are not producing desired outcomes. Also, children might be coping with their grief in unhealthy, yet effective ways. For example, a young teen might start experimenting with alcohol or drugs to relieve the stress of grief. Although this experimentation might be effective in temporarily pushing aside the pain, it is unhealthy behavior. The teen might find it helps in the short term, not fully understanding the long-term implications of such choices.

Professionals can work with children to identify healthy alternatives for coping with their grief. For example, some children cope with their grief through physical activity and sports. Other children cope by spending time with friends and having fun. Children often find comfort by talking with understanding people (their coach, a teacher, their parent, or a friend). They might seek reassurance and comfort from others, like a young child who crawls into a parent's lap and wants to be held when feeling sad. Children can also cope with grief in a healthy way by remembering the fun times they shared with the person who died. In addition, doing something nice for someone else or helping others in need can provide a positive feeling that helps children cope with their own difficulties (Table 6.2).

Table 6.2 Factors That Promote Health in Bereaved Children

Factor	How to Help
Positive parent–child relationship	Encourage parents to use an interactive, conversational style of communication, rather than leading with probing questions.
Expression and validation of grief	Provide parents with information about the types of reactions they might see in their children to normalize their understanding of their child's grief experiences.
A child's sense of control	Provide options during support sessions so children can choose. Encourage parents to provide choices for their children in the home and to validate their children's preferences.
Positive self-esteem	Work with children to set small achievable goals that result in small successes and help children problem solve challenging situations.
Healthy coping skills	Work with children to identify healthy ways to cope with their grief. Help children identify healthy alternatives to coping to replace potentially harmful ones.

SUMMARY

One of the primary purposes of bereavement support for children is to promote the health of children. Research shows that children who have a positive relationship with their parent or caregiver have the opportunity for expression and validation of their grief, have a sense of control over their own lives, have positive self-esteem, and have healthy ways of coping are better able to manage the challenges of grief (Haine et al., 2008). These elements are important for professionals to consider as they develop modes of helping and organize a safe space for children to be supported in their grief (Table 6.3).

Table 6.3 Healthy Ways to Cope With Grief
Talk about it.
Cry about it.
Write about it (free write, songs, poems, or letters).
Create art (paint, sculpt, mold, draw, or ceramics).
Do something physical (hike, run, walk, or play sports).
Listen to music.
Play music.
Create a memorial page on the computer.
Do volunteer work.
Read a book.
Build something.
Plant a tree.
Plant a garden.
Make a scrapbook.
Take photographs.
Spend time with family or friends.
Go to the cemetery.
Connect with others with a similar loss.
Go to the movies.
Spend time alone.

REFERENCES

Greeff, A. P., & Berquin, H. (2004). Resilience in families in which a parent has died. *American Journal of Family Therapy, 32*, 27–42.

Grollman, E. A. (1990). *Talking about death: A dialogue between parent and child.* Boston, MA: Beacon Press.

Haine, R. A., Ayers, T. S., Sandler, I. N., & Wolchik, S. A. (2008). Evidence-based practices for parentally bereaved children and their families. *Professional Psychology: Research and Practice, 39*, 113–121.

Haine, R. A., Wolchik, S. A., Sandler, I. N., Millsap, R. E., & Ayers, T. S. (2006). Positive parenting as a protective resource for parentally bereaved children. *Death Studies, 30*, 1–28.

Hurd, R. C. (1999). Adults view their childhood bereavement experiences. *Death Studies, 23*, 17–41.

Sandler, I. N., Wolchik, S. A., & Ayers, T. S. (2007). Resilience rather than recovery: A contextual framework on adaptation following bereavement. *Death Studies, 32*, 59–73.

Schuurman, D., & DeCristofaro, J. (2007). After a parent's death: Group, family and individual therapy to help children. In N. B. Webb (Ed.), *Play therapy with children in crisis* (pp. 173–196). New York, NY: Guilford Press.

Silverman, P. R., Weiner, A., & Elad, N. (1995). Parent-child communication in bereaved Israeli families. *Omega—Journal of Death and Dying, 31*, 275–293.

Worden, J. W. (1996). *Children and grief: When a parent dies.* New York, NY: Guilford Press.

Modes of Helping

I would urge professionals to take the time to listen well; to be patient and really develop relationships with the children they work with, so they can offer them the best support through this challenging time.

—*William Worden (an interview with Hospice Foundation of America)**

It is useful for professionals to have a variety of ways to help children explore their grief and adapt to the changes that grief has brought to their lives. As previously mentioned, grief often robs children of their sense of control over their own world. Professionals can empower children by providing a space in the support setting for children to make meaning of their loss, continue a connection to the deceased, and strengthen their ability to cope. This chapter explores some of the modes of helping that we have found to be effective over the years as we have provided support to bereaved children and their families.

FOSTERING MEANING-MAKING

The death of someone in a child's life shatters a child's assumptions and core beliefs about the world (Janoff–Bulman, 1992). Grieving children realize that life is not fair. They might come to realize that just because you are a "good person" does not mean that bad things will not happen to you. Bereaved children also learn early in life that you do not always have the control you thought you had over life events. The search for meaning arises out of the need to rebuild order in their lives. Children's sense of self is formed through the stories they tell about themselves. "Meaning-making" is an approach that you can use with individuals to help them reconstruct their personal narrative as they rebuild their sense of self (Neimeyer, 2009). The search for meaning is an important part of a child's adaptation to the new world brought about by his or her loss and is

**J. William Worden, PhD, ABPP., An Interview with Hospice Foundation of America, © Hospice Foundation of America.*

one of the primary ways the child works through his or her grief (Neimeyer, 2001). Schwartzberg and Janoff–Bullman (1991) found that people do better when they search for and find meaning, which in turn is related to less intense grief.

Finding meaning in the midst of suffering is a powerful tool that professionals can share with those under their care. In his book, *Man's Search for Meaning*, Viktor Frankl (1992) provides a framework for helping individuals to tell, reframe, and assign meaning to their own story. In this regard the professional offering support serves as a facilitator for a child to share and explore various aspects of his or her own story. It is important to note that meaning is never assigned to a child's story by the professional. Meaning can only be assigned by the storyteller.

The professional can act as a scribe, writing down the child's story, or supporting the child as he or she writes out his or her own story. Reframing can sometimes be a helpful tool as well. This is when the child, with the support of a professional, might evaluate the way he or she is looking at a particular event. The child might explore how he or she is interpreting the event and how this interpretation is impacting the child's grief. As children revisit particular aspects of this story, they often reframe some of their thinking. This is particularly true when they are able to share their story through talking, writing, or creative expression (art, music, etc.).

In addition to finding meaning in the midst of suffering, Frankl also outlined three ways people (including children) find meaning in their lives. First, children experience meaning in their lives through encountering other people in relationships. Our primary relationships help to form who we are. Relationships shape our way of thinking and being in the world and are strong bonds that we develop with other people in our lives. When someone in a child's life dies, the relationships the child has with surviving family and friends are an important part of the child's continued narrative. These relationships will help to shape grieving children into the people they are becoming. Also significant is the relationship they have with the deceased person. Though the bond with that person is strained because the person is no longer physically present, the impression of that person's life is still very much alive within the child. We discuss this continued relationship in the next section on continuing bonds. What is important to note here is that relationships are a primary source of our own personal meaning in life. As professionals we can encourage children to continue to build strong connections with the people in their lives. We can also provide helpful information and encouragement to the adults in children's lives to continue important connections, as these can be sustaining to children in their grief.

Second, children find meaning by encountering the world around them. This includes environments like their home, school, neighborhood, and community. Frankl asserted that meaning is found in the relationship we have with nature and exploring the natural world. In today's world, children's environments encompass nature less and less as a child's world consists of technology such as video games, television, cell phones, and computers. Though it is still unclear what effect the rise in technology will have on future generations, it is important to note that children today find meaning in these activities. At the same time, children thrive in environments where they can play, participate in arts and crafts activities, make believe, and interact with the natural world. Professionals can provide space for children to have these experiences in support group, individual support, and camp settings. Grief camps can be an ideal setting for children to work through their grief in a natural setting. Many grief camps are "unplugged," meaning that cell phones and video games are not permitted during the time that children are at camp. This allows children to connect to the natural world and to each other without the distraction of technology. Grief camps will be discussed further in the next chapter on support settings.

Finally, Frankl noted that we find meaning through our ability to be creative. This often manifests itself in our work or activities to which we apply ourselves and see results from our efforts. For children this can take the form of drawing pictures, painting, building forts out of sheets, or defeating a level on a video game. Professionals can help children to be creative by providing opportunities to participate in creative activities. These types of activities provide a context for making meaning out of their loss, but also provide an opportunity to connect with life and with one another.

Each of these activities—encountering others in relationships, encountering the world around us, and being creative—provides opportunity for children to tell their story, evaluate their own ideas, hear others tell their stories, and reframe their own stories as they make meaning out of their own loss (Figure 7.1).

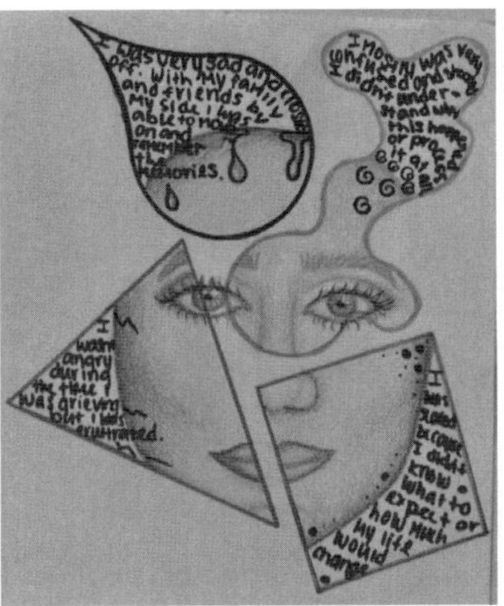

Figure 7.1 Artwork created by a teenager whose uncle died.

ENCOURAGING CONTINUING BONDS

As previously mentioned in Chapter 1, the common thinking in the early to mid-20th century was that one worked through grief by detaching oneself mentally and emotionally from the deceased person. The concept of "continuing bonds," as developed by Klass, Silverman, and Nickman (1996), stands in stark contrast to this idea that one must detach from a loved one in order to get better. Instead, continuing bonds asserts that grief is a transitional process in which one adjusts to the loss of the relationship with the deceased, while at the same time redefining and continuing the relationship in a different way. In this regard, professionals can support children by providing space for them to transition their relationship with the deceased to one of memories and thoughts, as opposed to a physical presence. This is another opportunity for professionals to meet children where they are, as it is common for children to connect with the deceased person in their own mind through conversations and thoughts about the person. Children are better able to manage the reality of the person's physical absence from their life when they are encouraged to remember the person who died and to do things to honor his or her memory.

Adjusting to the Loss of Relationship

As discussed in Chapters 1 and 2, children struggle to adapt to the many changes that the death of someone in their life brings. Not only do they miss the role that the person played in their lives, but they miss the physical presence of the person, as well. They will often long for the person who has died and grieve over their inability to interact with the person, to hear the person's voice, or to share conversation and experiences with that person. Children will sometimes try to avoid thinking about the person early on in their grief because when they do, it reminds them of their loss and it is painful. Yet, as children are given the opportunity to remember the person who died—although confronted with the stark reality of their absence—children are afforded the prospect of adjusting to the loss of the relationship. The support environment should allow space for children to remember the person who died, but professionals should be patient with children as they adjust to the loss of the relationship in their own time and at their own pace.

Redefining the Relationship

The reality is that a child's relationship with a person does not end when the person dies. We regularly encounter adults who had a parent die when they were children. They often report that they continue to think about, talk to, and feel a connection to their deceased loved one even as adults. Adapting the relationship with the deceased person to be one of memories and thoughts, as opposed to physical presence, is not an easy task for children. However, it is an important task for children as they redefine their relationship with the person who died. Professionals should provide activities in the support setting that help children to make this transition.

Continuing the Relationship

As the relationship continues with the deceased person, children might connect with the person in their mind through conversations, thoughts, and activities. This continued relationship is often very personal and many times children will not talk about it with other people. For example, children might imagine that their deceased parent is watching them when they are playing a sport or receiving an award. The notion that the deceased person is watching the child should come from the child, however, rather than being told that by another person. Children might imagine that their deceased parent is proud of them. They might ask this parent to help to steady their nerves when they are in a stressful situation. In this regard, they are continuing a relationship with the deceased person in their mind. This continued relationship can positively reinforce the child's sense of confidence and their belief in their ability to succeed (Figure 7.2).

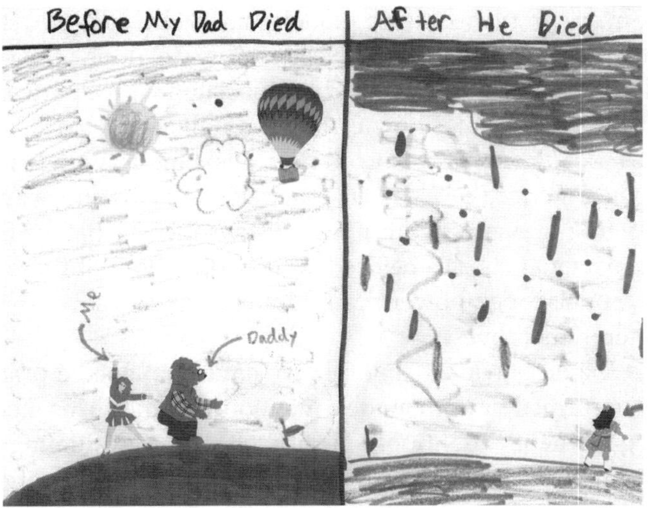

Figure 7.2 Artwork created by an older child whose dad died.

Honoring the Legacy of the Relationship

Honoring the legacy of the relationship is yet another way that children continue their bond with the person who died. They might dedicate a performance or some other type of venture to the deceased person. It is not unusual to see professional athletes point to the sky in reference to a deceased loved one after they score a touchdown, make a goal, or hit a homerun. Professionals can provide space in the support setting for children to create memorials for, dedicate activities to, and share stories about the person who died. It should never be assumed that children have fond feelings about the person who died. These activities should be made available as options for children in the support setting, but they should never be forced to participate in legacy-honoring activities.

PROMOTING PROBLEM SOLVING

Another powerful tool professionals have in supporting bereaved children is to offer a model for children to do problem solving. Professionals can provide children with a model to examine the variety of options available to them for reacting to the events occurring in their daily lives. The reality is that children often have limited impact on the many events in their lives, anything from big events like the death of a parent to minor events such as someone saying something insensitive to them. Providing children with strategies for problem solving affords them the opportunity to regain a sense of control over their world by reestablishing the belief that their choices matter.

There are many problem-solving models that might be employed. Cognitive behavioral therapy offers the "Think, Feel, Do" model (Ellis & Harper, 1961) in which one might evaluate one's thoughts associated with a particular event in one's life. One then evaluates how certain thoughts evoke particular feelings, which, in turn, leads one to act in certain ways. Similarly, in his book, *Seven Habits of Highly Effective People* (1989), Stephen Covey provides an alternative to simply reacting to events in our lives. Covey suggests that we first pause to consider our personal choices before taking action. Both of these approaches are effective models for empowering children to problem solve challenges that they encounter in their lives.

In our work with bereaved children, we have employed a practical model that has been informed by both models mentioned earlier. This model includes the following elements: identifying a difficult event, evaluating options for action, choosing an action, and taking action. The professional can use this model to walk children through the process of evaluating their options, choosing an option, and finally taking action, as opposed to simply reacting in the moment (see Figure 7.3). There are a variety of ways this can be employed in

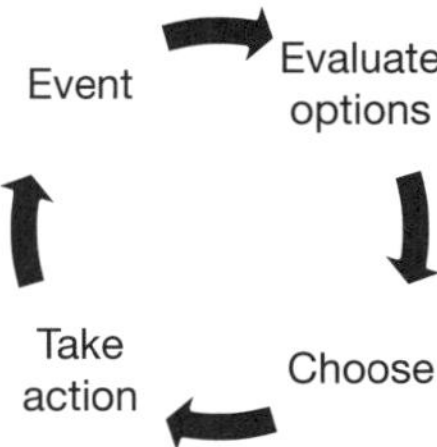

Figure 7.3 Problem-solving model.

both group and individual settings. In a group setting, a professional might ask the children in the group to identify some situations that have been particularly difficult for them since the death of their person. The group then selects one of the situations to be applied to the problem-solving model. In an individual setting, the professional asks the child to think of a situation that has been particularly challenging since the death. As a group, or one on one with a professional, children can go through the following steps.

Step One: Evaluating Options for Action

Professionals can explain to children that there are a variety of ways that children might react to events in their lives. As previously mentioned, there is no right or wrong way to react when grieving. Professionals should seek to normalize a child's experience. First, identify a particularly challenging situation. The more specific the details, the better. Then, whether one on one or in a group setting, professionals can help children identify various ways that they might react in given situations. It is important to allow the children to come up with their own ideas, rather than providing the options for them. There are many ways to accomplish this. Professionals might have children individually identify ideas and then share in a larger group discussion. Professionals might also take suggestions in open discussion with the entire group and then record these ideas on paper for all of the children to see. Either way, it is important that children are able to see that there are a variety of options for taking action in any given situation.

Step Two: Choosing an Action

After collecting a number of ideas about different responses to the situation, professionals should help children evaluate choosing an action. Choosing an action to an event is an important step. Choosing an action involves walking through the possible consequences of any particular response to a situation.

So children might select one of the options for action and then discuss what might be the result of applying this choice to the situation. You might do this with a number of the options before children select the particular action they will employ should this situation occur again. Identifying "choice" as a problem-solving step is also important because it once again emphasizes to children that choices matter.

Step Three: Taking Action

It is equally important for children to imagine themselves taking action, rather than just reacting to events in their lives. We have found that children will come back to group or counseling the next time and share about situations in which they employed the problem-solving model and chose to act, rather than react. When children are empowered to take action, they are able to establish a sense of control over their own world.

FACILITATING PERSPECTIVE BUILDING

Perspective-building activities are important because they provide children the opportunity to think about and evaluate their situation in light of new information. Children's perceptions are often restricted to their own limited experiences when it comes to understanding their grief, how that grief impacts their lives, and how to react in any given circumstance. Perspective-building activities allow children to expand and develop new constructs (schemas) that accommodate the new reality brought about by their loss. Perspective-building activities are also related to meaning-making and problem solving as they are a way children can evaluate and reframe key aspects of their own story.

One way professionals can help children build their perspective is to provide children with simple, easy-to-understand information about grief and common ways children are impacted by it. Children might feel like they are the only ones who feel like, or think like, they do. They might also think that they are the only people going through the same type of loss. Providing information about how grief impacts children and information about the types of losses children might experience can help to normalize children's feelings about their own situation. This is especially important for one-on-one counseling because children are not in a group setting with other children where they can relate to the stories of others.

Groups inherently provide the space for perspective building. When children are able to gather with other children going through a similar situation, they often feel comforted that they are not alone in their grief. The feeling that someone else understands what one is going through has a huge impact on a child's own sense of self-esteem. Groups also provide an opportunity for children to share about their grief experiences. As children hear the stories of others and about how others are dealing with their grief, they are encouraged that they can grieve and at the same time continue to live and thrive even in the midst of their grief.

There are also a variety of activities that professionals might use with children to help to build perspective. Gestalt developed a number of approaches that can be useful in the bereavement support setting. Often, children have unfinished business with the person who died. Unfinished business might be things they wish they had said that they did not say. It might also be something that they hoped their person would have said to them. It could involve regrets that they have about their last few interactions with the person who died. Children might feel the need to work through or express these types of thoughts and feelings to the deceased. Some examples of activities that help with unfinished business are having the child write a letter to the person who died, or having the child imagine what the person who died would say to him or her, and writing a letter from the person who died. For activity ideas, please refer to Chapter 9.

THE STRENGTH OF RITUALS

As previously mentioned, rituals provide a context for celebrating, commemorating, worshipping, and honoring. Rituals are often steeped in culture and tradition. They bring comfort and connection to people during both times of celebration and times of distress. After the death of someone, rituals offer a framework for some of the concepts presented previously, including meaning-making, continuing bonds, and perspective building. Rituals can be a powerful tool for professionals to use in the support setting as they can also establish predictable, familiar routines for group interactions, including openings, connecting activities, and closings (see Chapter 8).

Funerals are perhaps the most widespread end-of-life ritual throughout many societies and cultures. Funerals take on a variety of forms, from services of remembrance to celebrations of life. Typically, they reflect the culture of those leading and attending the service. The funeral provides the opportunity for the bereaved to find connection to others and to begin the process of adapting to their loss (Lucke, Gilbert, & Barrett, 2006). As professionals working with bereaved children, you will encounter parents and families who struggle with whether their children should attend the funeral or not. If the children do attend, parents often struggle with how much the children should be involved in the ceremony and planning.

Children should be offered the opportunity to both attend and participate in the funeral and end-of-life rituals with their family and community. Research indicates that children who attended funerals find them beneficial (Silverman & Worden, 1992). Also, families whose children are not permitted to attend the funeral are less well over time than children who are able to attend the funeral (Fristad, Cerel, Goldman, Weller, & Weller, 2001). Although it is helpful for children to attend funerals, it is important to prepare children for the funeral. A good process to suggest to families is for the parents or trusted adult to sit down with the children to prepare them. Children do better when they know what to expect. Preparing children for the funeral involves explaining to them the purpose for the funeral, what types of things they are likely to see at the funeral, and going over the planned schedule of events. If children do not want to attend the funeral, they should not be forced to do so. Appropriate arrangements should be made for children who do not want to attend.

If possible, children should be offered the opportunity to participate in the funeral in some way. This could also include being part of planning the funeral. Children are too often left out and even ignored during the funeral proceedings. This is a missed opportunity to engage children in the funeral ritual. Children might be encouraged to write a letter to the person who died, or asked if they have a special object they would like included in the casket. Children might be asked to write a few words to share about the person who died and what that person meant to their life. It is helpful to consider a number of ways children might participate and to give them choices. This will allow children to participate in the way that feels most comfortable to them.

Also, professionals should encourage families to assign a trusted adult to attend to the children during the funeral. This is an important part of preparing children for the funeral. This is particularly helpful for gatherings that might be lengthy like visitations. Children might be ready to go long before events are over. Assigning a trusted adult who does not have to stay for the entire event can alleviate worry by parents who might have responsibilities or need to stay. Some funeral homes today even have playrooms for children when they grow tired of the funeral events.

SUMMARY

The modes of helping mentioned earlier provide a basis for offering support to bereaved children and their families. These are strategies that we have employed in our work with bereaved children throughout our careers and we have found them to be effective ways for children to express their grief, explore strategies for coping with grief reactions, and adapt to the changes brought about by the death of someone in their lives. We encourage professionals to utilize these strategies when working with bereaved children and their families. Keep in mind that children should have a variety of choices and should never be forced to participate in any of these modalities. Instead, children should be invited to participate and be allowed to determine their own level of participation.

REFERENCES

Ellis, A., & Harper, R. A. (1961). *A guide to rational living*. Englewood Cliffs, NJ: Prentice-Hall.

Frankl, V.E. (1992). *Man's search for meaning: An introduction to logotherapy* (4th ed.). Boston, MA: Beacon Press.

Fristad, M. A., Cerel, J., Goldman, M., Weller, E. B., & Weller, R. A. (2001). The role of ritual in children's bereavement. *Omega—Journal of Death and Dying, 42*, 321–340.

Janoff–Bulman, R. (1992). *Shattered assumptions*. New York, NY: Free Press.

Klass, D., Silverman, S., & Nickman, S. (Eds.). (1996). *Continuing bonds: New understandings of grief*. Washington, DC: Taylor & Francis.

Lucke, G., Gilbert, R., & Barrett, R. K. (2006). *Death and religion in a change world*. New York, NY: Routledge.

Neimeyer, R. A. (Ed.). (2001). *Meaning reconstruction and the experience of loss*. Washington, DC: American Psychological Association.

Neimeyer, R. A. (2009). *Constructivist psychotherapy*. Washington, DC: Taylor & Francis.

Schwartzberg, S. S., & Janoff–Bulman, R. (1991). Grief and the search for meaning. *Journal of Social & Clinical Psychology, 10*, 270–288.

Silverman, P. R., & Worden, J. W. (1992). Children's reactions in the early months after the death of a parent. *American Journal of Orthopsychiatry, 62*, 93–104.

CHAPTER 8

Grief Support Settings for Bereaved Children

Anyone who does anything to help a child is a hero to me.

—Fred Rogers, Television Personality

CREATING A SAFE SPACE FOR SUPPORT

Creating a warm, accepting environment where children feel safe is an important component in providing support. This chapter discusses the characteristics of creating such a space for bereaved children. Professionals are advised about the elements of a safe environment and how to gain the trust of the children under their care. Foundational to this are the *five Universal Realities of Grief* and the implications of these on our interactions with children and how we provide the space they need to process their grief experiences.

Dimensions of Safe Space

Throughout this book we have suggested that professionals make space available for specific types of interventions and activities that support children in their grief. The space we provide for activities is just as important as the actual activities themselves. This section examines some of the necessary elements that constitute a safe space for children to express, process, and find support for their grief.

Physical Setting

A good place to start with a discussion of safe space is to look at the actual physical setting that will be used to provide support to bereaved children and their families. The physical setting reflects a message to families from the moment they arrive and throughout their experience in the support setting. From the colors of the walls to the setup of the rooms, it is important that the physical setting is warm, comfortable, and inviting to children. It is also important that the physical setting is reflective of hope, particularly for families facing very difficult times. For example, children's artwork, motivational posters, and displays of activities provide an environment that is nurturing and establishes a setting that is safe for children to express their grief.

The space should be conducive to the age and interests of the children attending support. For example, younger children might feel more comfortable sitting in chairs at tables that match their size. Furnishings for teenagers might consist of couches or more casual types of furniture, and décor might reflect generational norms of that particular age group. Beanbags arranged in a circle are also a consideration. It is also important that the space provides adequate confidentiality for children and their families and that the setting is large enough to accommodate the personal space of children and their families participating in counseling or support.

It is also important for the space to be inclusive of all children attending counseling. Artwork and images on posters and paintings should be multicultural. It is important for all children attending support to see themselves reflected in the images in the setting. For example, one bereavement center had a huge mural on the wall of the lobby of a beach scene. The picture was primarily of the natural landscape you might see at the beach with the exception of three small children. Two children were depicted as seemingly a Caucasian girl and boy, and a third child was depicted as an African American girl. One day, one of the board members approached the executive director and asked whether he could have a moment of his time. The board member took the executive director to the beach scene in the lobby and explained that growing up as an African American little boy, he never saw himself depicted in positive images or scenes. The board member suggested that the center further diversify the children on the beach so that children coming to counseling might see themselves in the images. So professionals should consider how the images, décor, and other aspects of the physical setting reflect diversity and inclusiveness. This can be important to providing a space that is comfortable to *all* children attending support.

People

The people within the physical setting are an important part of creating a safe space for children and their families. These include the paid staff and volunteers—from those providing support and counseling to those answering the phone and greeting families as they arrive. From the very first contact with parents and their children, there should be a spirit of compassion and empathy regarding their situation.

Just as the physical setting can reflect warmth, hope, and comfort, so, too, should the staff and volunteers working with families reflect these characteristics. This is true for whatever type of support setting you might be providing. For example, in our individual and family counseling practices, our physical space was arranged so that both children and their parents would feel comfortable sharing and participating. Many individual counseling settings can have an institutional feel to them and families arrive without being greeted because of a lack of reception staff. It is important in the case of bereavement support that the setting is comfortable, reflecting more homelike settings than that of a medical office. It is optimal if children and adults are greeted as they arrive because children and adults are often nervous about their first visit. A kind greeting from a compassionate person as they arrive can go a long way to ease some of this apprehension.

The Role of Staff and Volunteers in Creating a Safe Space

Staff and volunteers should be respectful of a child's personal space, should be nonjudgmental, and should be comfortable being around children who are grieving. These sentiments might seem obvious, but a reminder is important because these elements are not always followed, as it can be challenging at times for staff and volunteers to separate their own personal loss experience from their care for bereaved children and their families. This is also challenging because we all share the human experience that people we love will die. Striking a balance between personal, compassionate care, and professional boundaries is necessary to protect the support environment. This is discussed further in Chapter 10.

Respect for Personal Space

It is important to keep in mind that grief belongs to the child who is grieving and that the child should be given the space to participate in counseling as he or she is comfortable doing. Children have to invite us into their world and there might be parts of their grief that they are not comfortable sharing. Because grief is not a problem we are trying to solve, or an illness we are treating, we can be patient with children and their families as they are adapting to their new reality. Seasoned staff and volunteers can advocate for children and their families by modeling good boundaries for newer staff and volunteers supporting bereaved children.

Nonjudgment

Bereaved children and their families often come to the support setting having been judged by extended family, friends, or even peers. Therefore, providing a setting in which children and families do not feel or perceive judgment is important. All of us, even professionals, have biases. Being aware of our own predispositions and preconceived ideas is important so that our own biases do not intrude into the support setting. This is essential to providing a safe space for children and their families to express their grief. When children can express their grief in an environment free from judgment, they are more likely to open up and process aspects of their grief that they may not feel comfortable sharing in other settings.

Comfortable Being Around Bereaved Children

Professionals who intend to work with bereaved children should take some time for self-reflection about their comfort level being with bereaved children. Some children are energetic and tend to move from one activity to another. Others might be more quiet, reserved, and slow to open up. Both of these types of personalities present their own challenges for adults providing support. Children can sometimes try our patience and adults working with children should have a comfort level with diverse personalities, energy levels, and varied dispositions. Bereaved children specifically, when they feel comfortable enough to share, will disclose details about their loss and personal feelings about their grief that might be difficult to hear. For some adults, it can be difficult to hear children share their grief and personal pain.

Communication Techniques and Building Rapport

The best place to start with a discussion about communicating and building rapport with children is to start by getting to know the children under your care. How we build rapport and communicate with children might vary based on the personality and preferences of the children with whom we are working. Some children are more quiet than others, their interests may vary, and the ways they feel most comfortable in the world might be wide ranging. Whether we are working with children in a group or in an individual setting, observing and listening is a good first step to opening up communication and building a trusting relationship. For example, during an intake with a child in an individual counseling session, you might prepare an overview of what the child can expect from week to week while attending counseling, and provide an initial activity for the child to complete, rather than sitting with the child asking questions or trying to get the child to talk. Professionals might find that as they are able to build rapport and trust with a child, the child will open up more and more from week to week. The following are examples of communication techniques that help to build trust and rapport with children under your care.

Active and Reflective Listening

Active listening involves reflecting back to children what you hear them saying. For example, a child might say, "When my dad died, in the beginning I was really confused about what was happening." A professional might respond with, "I see, you were confused about what was happening." This reassures the child that you are hearing what he or she is saying and offers the opportunity for the child to then share more insight into what it was that he or she was confused about. Also, by reflecting back what you are hearing, it helps to lessen the number of probing questions you are asking a child. Children respond better when they feel as though they are not under a microscope, but instead are sharing freely with someone who is actively listening to what they are saying. Active listening enables the child to direct the conversation, whereas probing questions redirect the conversation to where the professional wants things to go. The ideal is for the child to direct the conversation. This is how we get to know the child and the child's perspective on his or her experiences.

Letting Children Lead in Play

Children are the experts of their own world. This is particularly true when they are playing. Children will be drawn toward those activities with which they feel most comfortable. Professionals have a great opportunity to connect with children by following children in their play. Children feel safe sharing and interacting when professionals follow their lead, prompting as they play. Professionals should provide children with options of what they might do. Once they choose an activity, join them in that activity. There is no better way to connect with children than to follow them in their play.

Being Present With Children While Completing an Activity

Children love it when adults give them attention. It is not unusual to hear a child exclaim, "Watch this!" or to have them approach you and say, "Look what I did." Children want to feel like someone "gets them" and that what they are doing matters. Because of this, it is important that professionals working with bereaved children are present with children while they are completing an activity. They can have a conversation with them about the activity, or even do the same activity next to the child. Professionals should use caution asking questions like, "What are you making?" or "Is that a picture of your dad?" It is more effective to make observations like, "I see you are using a lot of red in your picture," or "I noticed that you are using blue yarn to make your craft." This lets children know that you are watching what they are doing without assigning any meaning or making any assumptions. This allows children to share as much or as little as they want with the professional about what the activity means or represents.

Process

Children thrive in environments that are predictable and where they know what is expected of them. For this reason, an organized process, and how we go about providing counseling and support, is imperative to creating a safe space for bereaved children and their families. The process includes informed consent, established ground rules, curriculum, schedule, and planned activities. The process should allow room for personal expressions of grief. It is also important for the process to be age appropriate. For example, young children might need to move from one activity to another more quickly than older children. The process should also offer room for a variety of activities and options that empower children to participate in the way they feel most comfortable. Keep in mind that expressions of grief are not something that only happens through talking. Children express their grief through play, writing, artwork, and other activities. It is also important that the group or session begin and end on time. This helps to support an environment that is predictable.

Ground Rules and Expectations

The professional is the overseer of the process. It is the professional's role to facilitate, maintain, and protect the process in order to preserve the integrity of the support setting. The ground rules are the shared contract that the professional has with the counseling or support participant(s), whether in a group or individual setting. These ground rules set the expectations for participation and behavior in the group. For example, in a group setting a ground rule might be that we do not talk when someone is telling his or her story. The facilitator is responsible for holding participants accountable to follow this agreed-upon rule and to intervene if members of the group are showing a lack of respect to another group member. This helps to maintain the balance in the group so that children know the space is safe for them to openly share from their perspective.

Measurement and Evaluation

Measuring the impact of the services on the lives of children provides important information to professionals on the effectiveness of their programs. Feedback from children and their parents can help inform continued care, ideas for further development of programming, and needed improvements in service delivery. There are two levels of measurement that a professional might use to evaluate his or her services. The first level of measurement is to ascertain satisfaction with the services provided. This might include questions about children and their families' experience during the intake process, the timing and frequency of sessions, or satisfaction with staff and volunteers. This information is important to continue to organize the structure and type of support offered.

The second level of measurement is to measure the impact of services on the lives of the children participating in the grief support services. This might include a pre- and posttest evaluation containing questions regarding a child's grief. For example, the pretest might include questions about a child's behavior. There could be questions about new challenges that the child has had since the death. We recommend that professionals use a similar format to provide an evaluation periodically throughout the time in support to benchmark progress, or at the end of their time attending support. Both levels of measurement can be combined into one document or handled separately. It is important that professionals measure the services being provided in whatever format works best for their setting. Otherwise, professionals are missing a huge opportunity to evaluate the effectiveness of their services and how those services impact the lives of children.

Content

If the process is the structure, format, and schedule of the group, the content of the session is the subject matter being discussed. Although the professional is the overseer of the process, the content is primarily provided by the participants in the counseling or support setting. *In other words, the subject matter is child driven and child led.* Bereaved children and their parents each have their own personal grief they are bringing with them into the setting. The support setting should provide space for telling the story, sharing concerns, posing questions, and expressing grief that the participants are dealing with at that time. Providing a structured space for them to openly express and explore their grief, the challenges grief brings, and ideas for coping with their grief is paramount to providing a safe space for support.

As discussed previously, grief is a personal experience and belongs to the griever. Professionals should protect the environment by providing space for children to share whatever their grief might look like at that moment and the issues that might be causing them distress. At the same time, grief is also a shared experience and it is important for children to be able to relate to those providing support. In this regard, both the professional and bereaved child might supply content to the support setting, but the space must allow for the child to openly share from his or her perspective. Self-awareness is an important component for professionals as they find the balance between identifying with the children they are supporting and allowing the children participating in support to supply the subject matter being processed.

TYPES OF SUPPORT SETTINGS FOR BEREAVED CHILDREN

Grief support and counseling are available for children and families in many places in the world. It is offered in a variety of settings from groups to individual and family counseling. In this section we take a closer look at specific settings and explore special considerations for providing grief support in each of these settings. As discussed in the previous section, creating a safe space in each of the following support settings is critical to effective delivery of grief support services to bereaved children.

Individual Support

Individual support for children is provided by a variety of professionals, including clergy, therapists, child life specialists, social workers, and health care workers, to name a few. Because of this, there are a variety of theoretical approaches to providing individual support, from counseling and therapy to strictly supportive, companioning models. Whatever the setting might be, there are some specifics that apply and some special considerations that should be taken into account when providing support individually to children and their families.

Personalized Care

Each person's grief journey is unique to that person's own situation. Individual and family counseling provide a context to offer more personalized support to children and their families. Professionals providing individual support have an opportunity to work with bereaved children and their families to better understand how the death of someone in their lives has impacted individuals within the family and the family unit as a whole. Care can then be personalized to support the individual needs of children, as well as to provide opportunities for families to support one another. Professionals are able to facilitate interactions between children and their parents, problem solve specific challenges within the home, and tailor support that addresses specific issues to that family.

Informed Consent

Within the field of grief support services, there is a distinction between grief support and grief counseling. Some counselors are licensed and some are not. There is also a distinction between mental health counseling and bereavement counseling. Because there are a variety of ways to refer to the services and to deliver individual support, it is important that professionals are clear with individuals and families about their credentials, what type of support they are providing, and the limitations of that support. This information should be provided both verbally and in writing during the first session with the family. This provides an up-front understanding with families regarding the type, extent, and scope of services being provided.

Peer Support Groups

Peer support groups offer unique opportunities to provide a safe space for children to interact with other bereaved children and experience support (Schuurman, 2014). Peer support groups might be facilitated by professionals or volunteers, or a combination of both. Peer support groups are offered in a variety of settings and might be open and ongoing, or closed and short term. It is important to note that providing a concurrent group for parents of bereaved children that meets separately during the same time as the children's support group is helpful (Schuurman & DeCristofaro, 2010). This provides an opportunity for parents to find support and connection. When parents are having their needs met and learning ways to be helpful to their children in the home, children fare better. There are a number of key elements of group support that should be considered in providing peer support groups. These considerations have implications on how peer support groups are offered and how services are delivered (Figure 8.1).

Group Format

Grief support groups for children come in a variety of formats and many different shapes and sizes. Open-ended and ongoing groups typically allow group members to start anytime throughout the year, whereas closed and time-limited groups most likely have parameters around when group members can begin a group. The duration of the group can differ depending on the individual or organization that is offering the group. An ongoing group might be offered throughout the year with no set number of sessions. Closed, time-limited groups will typically be offered for a specific number of sessions (8- or 12-week sessions). Depending on the format, some groups might have a curriculum that they follow, whereas others might not. Sometimes groups are formatted

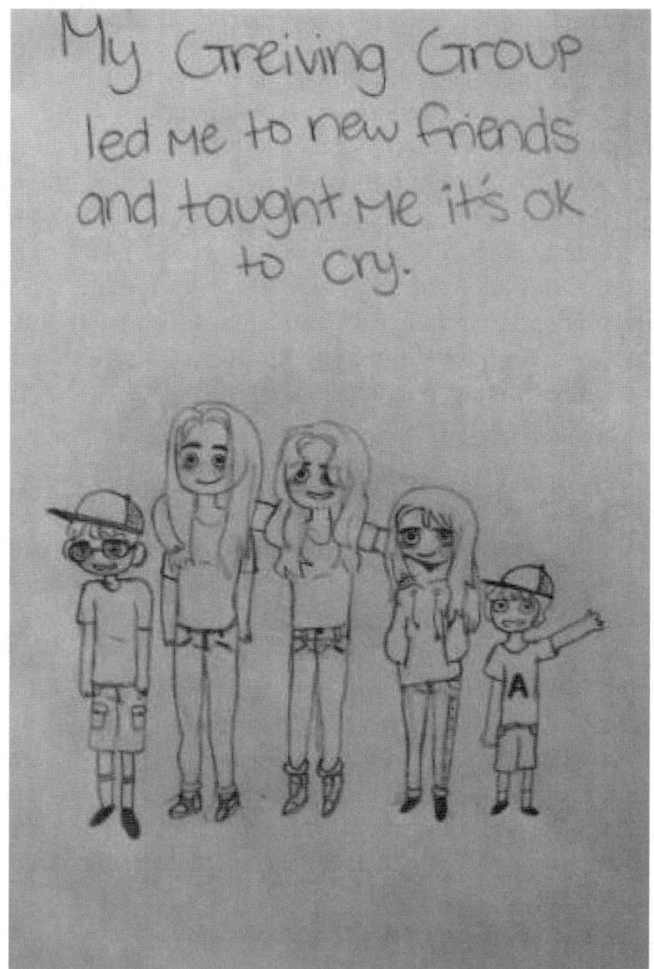

Figure 8.1 Artwork created by a teenager whose dad died.

based on the type of loss and who died. An example of this would be a support group for children who have had someone close to them die by suicide.

Intake Process and Screening

There are important components to the intake process that help to maintain a safe space in the group environment for all participants. These include screening participants for appropriateness for the group and establishing an orientation process to prepare attendees for what to expect in regard to the group process. For example, in our work with groups, we do not provide the date, time, or location details because we want to screen participants for group readiness and group appropriateness. When a grief group is advertised, the public might interpret the purpose of the group in a variety of ways. Parents might think the group is for any child grieving any type of loss (divorce, incarcerated parent, etc.). Further, some children and families might be dealing with issues outside the scope of what the group offers. For example, a parent might bring a child to a grief support group because of problem behaviors the parent is seeing in the child. Though there may be a loss history, screening might uncover that the problem behaviors are a result of something other than grief. Screening can help to alleviate this type of confusion and provide the opportunity to offer appropriate referrals.

Screening also allows the opportunity to orient potential group members to the process. Having a separate orientation meeting with families (whether individually or in a group) provides the opportunity to explain how the group works, go over ground rules for participating in group, and provide a snapshot of what to expect from the group. It also gives the opportunity for children and families to visit the physical space. This helps children feel more comfortable about attending their first night of group. In addition, they have the chance to meet staff or volunteers who will be there to greet them. If the orientation happens with a group of new potential members, they have the opportunity to meet other children who will be attending the group as well.

Structure and Flow of Group

The schedule and flow of group is important so children know what to expect from week to week. Group structure provides rituals that occur consistently in each group meeting. This familiarity and structure are comforting and offer predictability to children participating in the group. This helps to alleviate some of the stress of the unknown. The Dougy Center for Grieving Children has created a group model (1995) that has been adopted and adapted by bereavement support programs across the world. The following is the basic structure and flow of the group model created by The Dougy Center. There are a number of ways to structure and run peer support groups for children. We have found this format provides the necessary elements that create a safe space for children to share openly, while offering a variety of options.

Opening Circle

It is helpful for children to have a structured time during the beginning of group for introductions and checking in. The opening circle begins the safe space for the group. The ritual of the opening circle establishes a clear beginning to group time. It is important to establish a consistent routine to the opening circle and stick with this routine from week to week. This provides predictability for children, which, as mentioned previously, is important to establishing a safe space for children.

For the opening circle, have children sit in a circle. Depending on your setting, you might have limited seating options. If you have the ability to be creative, you might use beanbags, small chairs, or even big pillows. The more child friendly and comfortable you can make it, the better. The leader then welcomes the children to the group and takes a minute or 2 to explain the purpose of the group, what to expect during their time together, and to go over the ground rules. Ground rules should be simple and easy for kids to remember. Some examples of ground rules might be (a) the option to pass and not share, (b) to keep things confidential (what is said here stays here), (c) do not interrupt or talk over someone who is sharing, (d) no putdowns are allowed, and (e) a child must be with an adult at all times.

The leader then explains that everyone will have an opportunity to introduce himself or herself. Typically, this includes the child's name, age, who died, and how the person died. Many groups will have a "talking stick" or other symbolic object that is passed around from one group member to another. Whoever holds the "talking stick" has the floor and should have the attention of others in the group. The opening circle might conclude with this basic introduction, or leaders might opt to do another go around to allow another opportunity for children to freely share. Open-ended groups are more likely to have new children join the group on an ongoing basis than closed groups. Leaders can vary the format of the opening circle to meet the needs of their particular group, depending on whether the group uses an open or closed format.

Activity Time

After the opening circle this model provides for a time for kids to participate in a planned activity for that night. The activity might be themed to one of the factors that promote health in bereaved children. For example, an activity might be selected that offers the opportunity for children to express their grief and what they are currently going through. Depending on the number of staff or volunteers available, leaders might offer a couple of activity options for children in a single night. Keep in mind that activity content is most effective when it comes from the children in the group. Leaders might take note of emerging themes from group and one-on-one conversations to plan future activities. After the activity is completed, allow children the option to share their activity with the group. Children may also pass and not share their activity; it is completely up to them. In the group, facilitators are encouraged to point out common themes and to make connections between children. For more information on activities, please see Chapter 9.

Free Time/Snack Time

After activity time, it is helpful to offer a variety of options for children to have free time to play, draw, make believe, and interact with one another and the adult staff and volunteers. Though this is "free time," there are still structure and preplanned options from which the children might choose. Ground rules should still be emphasized and children should be held accountable to these agreed-upon boundaries. The options you are able to offer children will vary based on your space. The goal is to be as creative as you can to provide a variety of areas for play to occur. Some examples of spaces you might provide are (a) an artwork station; (b) a puppet or acting station; (c) a big-energy area with balloons or balls; (d) a play area with toy cars, toy dolls, houseware items; or (e) a crafts area. Again, whatever space you have, be creative and provide as much variety as possible. At the end of free time, it is helpful to offer a small snack to the children before moving to closing circle.

Closing Circle

Just as opening circle opens up the safe space, the closing circle provides a distinct ending to your time together. Closing circle offers the opportunity for children to share about their time together during that group session. Using a similar "go around" format from opening circle, the leader might ask the children who would like to share about their experience in group. This is also a good time to allow children to ask questions of the group. Once children have had an opportunity to share, the leader then leads the group in a closing ritual. A closing ritual should be established and should be consistent from week to week. This can be something simple like going around the room and everyone sharing one word that describes their time together.

Group Frequency and Size

How often your group meets might vary based on the number of staff and volunteers you have available. Typically, open-ended groups meet either biweekly or monthly, whereas closed-ended, short-term groups might meet weekly. In deciding upon group frequency, keep the structure of the group in mind and what it will take to provide a safe space for children each time you meet. For start-up groups, we suggest that you begin meeting monthly so you can establish a consistent format, collect activity ideas, and orient yourself to the process.

The size of the group is also dependent on the number of staff and volunteers you have available. During free time it is ideal to have no more than two children for every one adult. We would recommend not going over three children for every one adult at the most. This provides opportunity for children to interact with adults and share in a more one-on-one setting. With teens and older children the ratio might be higher as they will interact more easily with one another during activity and free time. The size of the group also matters when it comes to the opening and closing circles. We recommend not exceeding more than 12 to 15 individuals in any one group. When you reach this size, it is time to consider offering another group. You might divide groups based on age. This will help with the flow of opening and closing circles. You might have these smaller groups participate in opening and closing circles together and then come together during free time. Again, this is all dependent on your space and number of adults available.

Encouraging Participation and Minimizing Isolation

Groups will have a variety of types of personalities and a variety of types of losses. It is the facilitator's role to create a space for children to feel comfortable sharing and interacting with one another, while at the same time respecting these important differences. There are a number of ways facilitators can encourage participation and minimize isolation in a group setting. First, allow time and space for the child to get to know you and the other group members. Many times, the opening circle provides the ideal setting for this. As children hear the names, ages, and the types of loss everyone has experienced, they will often make connections and feel more comfortable participating themselves. Introduce yourself to children and introduce them to other children in the group with whom they might feel a rapport. This will help to foster trust, which often leads to group participation.

Another way to encourage participation is to allow children to choose the ways they feel most comfortable participating in the group. Having the rule that a child does not have to share if he or she does not want to helps to establish this precedent and empowers children to feel like they have a say in how they will participate. As previously mentioned, reestablishing a sense of control in a child's life is important to the child's own health and personal outlook. We have found that when children are given the option to participate in the ways they feel most comfortable, in time, they begin to open up and trust the leaders and other participants (Figure 8.2).

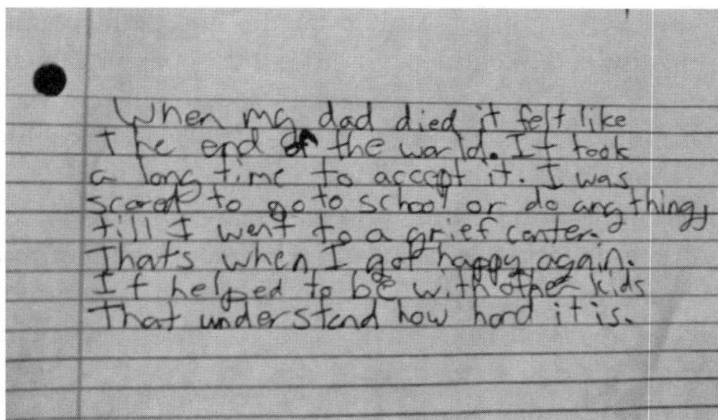

Figure 8.2 Created by a preteen whose dad died.

Grief Camps

In addition to individual support and peer support groups, grief camps are another setting that provides support to bereaved children. Grief camps allow children to process their grief in an environment that is different than the support that they are receiving at home or in school. Clute and Kobayashi (2013) found that grief camps are an effective means of helping grieving children cope with their loss. Camps can be single day or multiday and are similar to peer support groups with regard to the group dynamics. Camps provide a setting that allows for more opportunities for children to interact with one another in settings often unavailable during peer support groups. For example, camps typically offer swimming, canoeing, nature hikes, and similar activities that are available in an outdoor setting. Camps also offer children a large amount of intensive time with other children and have a unique healing component (McClatchey & Wimmer, 2012). At camp, children are able to explore deeper parts of their grief, their stories, and their perspectives with one another and build bonds with other children who have had similar experiences.

Grief Support in Schools

Another setting where children encounter and grapple with death is at school. Ideally, schools can provide a safe environment for children to receive grief support. Schools generally have a predictable schedule with structured activities and routines that children find comforting. Rules and boundaries are typically clearly spelled out so that children know what is expected of them. Normally, teachers strive to nurture and care for the children in their classrooms. School counselors and school administrators typically provide the guidance children and their families need. Though the primary purpose of school is to provide education to children, school officials often end up doing so much more. When a child has had someone in his or her life die, grief reactions often manifest themselves when the child is at school. Further, the death of a student or school staff member might necessitate a response from the school and support to children in the school setting. Here are a few considerations for school settings and suggestions about how to help children in this setting.

Supporting Children in the School After the Death of a Student, Teacher, or Staff Member

The death of a student, teacher, or staff member can have a profound impact on surviving students and school staff alike. It is important for schools to have a plan for responding to these types of situations in order to protect the integrity of the school setting. As previously mentioned, the school environment often provides a predictable, safe environment where children understand what is expected of them. It is important that schools preserve this setting, while at the same time acknowledge the loss everyone has experienced and offer opportunities for expression of grief. Throughout our careers, we have been called to schools to provide support after a death. There are a number of things schools can do to acknowledge the death, support children and faculty, and protect the integrity of the school setting.

Acknowledge the Life of the Person Who Died and Notify Students, Faculty, and Parents

When someone dies, it is important that the school acknowledges the life of the person who died. If there is a death that affects the school, students, faculty, staff, and parents must be notified. If a student has died, the first step in acknowledging the death is to reach out to the family of the student. We have often been asked by school officials after a death whether they should contact the family and, if so, when? Sometimes, school officials worry that they are being intrusive by reaching out to the family immediately after the death. It has been our experience that families are typically receptive to being contacted, especially when the purpose is to offer condolences and support. It is appropriate for school staff to contact families whether a student or a staff member dies. In the case of a child's death, most parents welcome hearing from the school, especially because this is where their child spent most of his or her time during the week. This is also true when it is a staff member who dies. Families typically appreciate hearing from the school where a loved one worked and spent so much time. When school officials reach out to grieving families, they are modeling helpful behavior that students and faculty alike can emulate.

Contacting families after a death also provides an opportunity for schools to open communication with families. This, in turn, helps school officials to be able to clarify information about the death and to find out how the family would like others to be notified. Misinformation and rumors can quickly spread after a death, especially with social media and smartphones. Schools can help by providing accurate information and setting an example of how to react after someone dies. It is recommended that school officials have a written statement for school leadership, counselors, and teachers. This helps to provide talking points when school staff interact with children. It is also important that the school notify students and faculty about the death. It is best if faculty can be notified as a group in a staff meeting either before or after school. It is also recommended that students and faculty be offered support when they are notified of the death. Some students and staff might be closer to the person who died than others, but this does not mean that those who were not as close will have less severe reactions.

When possible, we recommend notifying students about a death in the classroom setting. Classrooms offer a smaller, more contained setting. Classrooms typically develop their own culture and routines based on the personalities of the students and the teacher. Teachers can provide a stable, compassionate presence for their students as they are processing the death. It is helpful if teachers have an activity to do with children after they are notified of the death. This gives teachers an opportunity to discuss the death with the children in their classroom and also to give the children an outlet to work through what they are feeling. One activity we recommend for this setting is to have children make homemade condolence cards to be sent to the family. In this case, teachers can explain that it is customary to express one's thoughts and support to the family of the person. When possible, schools should provide assistance to teachers who might need additional help with notifying students or discussing the death with them. Local mental health professionals, chaplains, and others who work with children are typically willing to come into the school and provide additional support.

Finally, it is also important to notify parents about the death of a student or faculty member. This can be done by sending a note home with students that includes information about who died and how the school intends to support students in the wake of the death. Sending a letter home helps to lessen the number of phone calls schools receive. Letters can also help parents prepare for supporting their children in the home. In addition to the notification letter, schools can also include a handout about supporting children at home.

Many local mental health counselors have helpful information that could be reproduced and distributed to students after a death.

Provide an Option for Support Outside of the Classroom

Teachers should be encouraged to return the classroom to normal functioning after acknowledging the death and giving students the opportunity to express condolences to the family of the person who died. Most of the students in the classroom will be able to return to a normal classroom schedule. We do, however, advise that teachers give consideration to what has happened when testing or giving grades during the immediate time surrounding the death. Although many of the children in the classroom will return to a normal schedule, there will be some children who are not able to focus or return to their schoolwork. This might be for a variety of reasons. It could be that a child knew the person who died. Another possibility is that the death reminds a child of his or her own grief over the death of someone in the child's own family. Whatever the reason, it is helpful for schools to set up an option for children to seek support outside of the classroom.

In the days immediately following the death, we recommend that schools provide a safe place for students to be supported. This could be in a group or individual setting. We have found the library to be a good place for this type of gathering. Libraries are often calm, quiet settings with tables that can be conducive to offering helpful activities to children. This space should be staffed with counselors, chaplains, or other supportive people. It is important for these individuals to be trained to provide support to students in this situation. These individuals do not need to give a lot of advice, but should be there to sit with children while they complete activities and to be a supportive presence while the students express their grief.

After a death, school staff should make outside referrals to students, as necessary. In some cases, children who are dealing with other life difficulties might take advantage of this opportunity and come for additional support. Once children have had an opportunity to interact with others, participate in additional activities, and express their grief, school professionals should encourage children to return to their classroom with the understanding that if they need additional support, they should notify their teacher. Children should be allowed to come to the support setting as often as they like, but then they should be encouraged to return to class. This transition back into the normal classroom routine is important.

As we have noted, schools should acknowledge the life of the person who died, share honest information with the students and faculty, provide support both within and outside the classroom, and continue a normal classroom schedule. When this is done, students and faculty are able to feel supported while at the same time they glean the benefit of the stable, safe environment that the school setting provides. It is recommended that professionals supporting bereaved children should reach out to build relationships with school personnel before a death happens. Outside professionals can provide much-needed support to schools during these types of crisis situations.

Advice for Teachers in the Classroom

It is not unusual for teachers to have students in the classrooms who are grieving the death of someone in their family. Many times teachers will not be aware that someone has died, though sometimes parents will notify the school. Over the years, we have had countless teachers ask for advice on how to react to these students in the classroom. Teachers wonder whether they should acknowledge that they know about the death and offer their support, or whether they should wait until the child brings it up. These questions stem from concern for the well-being of the child. They also stem from not wanting to say the wrong thing and making the situation more difficult for the child.

Our advice to teachers in the classroom is that acknowledging a student's loss is acceptable. For example, a teacher may say to a student, "I heard about your dad's death and want you to know that I care about you. If you find yourself having a difficult time during class, you can let me know." We would recommend keeping it simple and avoiding giving advice or saying things to try to make the situation better like, "It will be okay," or "It will get better in time." The best thing teachers can do is to create a classroom environment that is safe and predictable, while at the same time showing compassion to the needs of the students under their care.

Holding Grief Support Groups During School Hours

Ongoing or short-term grief groups during school hours are growing in popularity today. This has happened for a number of reasons. Some children don't have the ability to access services outside of school and a school group might be their only way to receive grief support. Another factor is that schools are finding the need for additional support for the students, especially after the death of a student or member of the staff. It has been our experience that school settings are not always the most conducive to support. Some schools request that support be provided outside of school hours, allowing students to maintain a normal school schedule during school hours. This is not always possible. Some students will not receive any formalized support unless it is offered during school hours. In the case of in-school support, we offer the following recommendations.

First, the person providing support should always close the support time with a transitional activity or information that grounds children and prepares them to go back to class. As is true in any support setting, there should be some sort of ritual that helps to transition children from reflecting on their loss to moving back into a classroom setting and concentrating on their studies. This can be challenging in the school setting because time for groups is often limited to less than an hour. Second, it is important that students be given the option of participating or not. Attendance with the group should be optional and come in the form of an invitation, rather than a requirement.

SUMMARY

As professionals, we have the opportunity to provide a safe space for children to openly express their grief and to find support and understanding. The physical space, the processes we use, and the people providing the support all play an important role in establishing space that is safe for children. Likewise, the ability for children to contribute input or content to that space is paramount in establishing an environment that is supportive and comfortable to them. Support can be provided in an individual, group, or camp format. Each of these formats offers unique opportunities for supporting children and their families. Further, individual support and groups might be provided in a variety of settings, including schools, churches, or community support settings. The ideas and suggestions provided in this chapter can be adapted by professionals to work within any setting in which they might be supporting bereaved children.

REFERENCES

Clute, M. A., & Kobayashi, R. (2013). Are children's grief camps effective? *Journal of Social Work in End-of-Life & Palliative Care, 9*, 43–57.

McClatchey, I., & Wimmer, J. S. (2012). Healing components of a bereavement camp: Children and adolescence give voice to their experience. *Omega—The Journal of Death and Dying, 65*, 11–32.

Schuurman, D. L. (2014). Support groups for adolescents. In K. J. Doka & A. S. Tucci (Eds.), *Living with grief: Helping adolescents cope with loss.* Washington, DC: Hospice Foundation of America.

Schuurman, D. L., & DeCristofaro, J. (2010). Principles and practices of peer support groups and camp-based interventions for grieving children. In D. Balk & C. Corr (Eds.), *Children's encounters with death, bereavement, and coping* (pp. 359–372). New York, NY: Springer Publishing.

C H A P T E R 9

Activities That Engage Children

You can discover more about a person in an hour of play than in a year of conversation.

—*Plato*

It is paramount for professionals working with bereaved children to provide activities and opportunities for a child to explore his or her grief experience. Activities can provide insight to the professional about the child, the family prior to the death, and how the death has impacted the child's environment. If the child is comfortable sharing the activities with the parent, this can be helpful to the child's parents or caregivers so they can better understand the child's grief as they attempt to help their child at home. This chapter describes some things to keep in mind when planning activities for children and provides samples of activities that can be used with children in a support or counseling setting.

CONSIDERATIONS FOR SELECTING ACTIVITIES FOR CHILDREN

The Age or Maturity Level of Children

Young children are very literal in their interpretation of the world around them. Because of this, professionals should consider avoiding the use of too many metaphors to describe or talk about grief as part of activities used with younger children. On the other end of the spectrum, preteens and teenagers are often thinking about their grief and loss in very different ways than younger children. Preteens and teens often find support through interactive dialogue and activities that allow them to work together as a group. Professionals can also make a few material changes to activities and get a better response from preteens and teenagers. For example, for drawing activities, rather than using standard-sized paper, cut butcher paper to the size of a larger canvas. Rather than use crayons or markers, provide colored chalk as an option. These small changes will make the activity feel less "child-like" to teens and elicit a more positive response and willingness to participate.

Time Needed to Complete the Activity

Children, particularly younger children, have a short attention span. This includes their ability to sit with one activity for an extended length of time. Also, activities might lose their effectiveness if children do not have enough time to complete them before the allotted time. Professionals should consider the length of time needed to complete a planned activity and make sure that the schedule permits time for the activity to be completed. One exception to this is in an individual counseling setting. In this type of setting, children can focus on an activity for a little longer because of the individual attention being received. But, even in this setting, every child has a limit on how long he or she can stay with one activity before losing interest. As mentioned previously, there should be a variety of options for children in a support or counseling setting. Professionals should pay attention to children's engagement with an activity and be prepared to offer other options or to allow children to finish activities at a later time if they seem to be losing interest.

The Feasibility of the Activity

This might seem to be an obvious consideration, but it is worth noting that activities should be able to be finished and activities should be supportive of children. Professionals should complete the activity themselves prior to using it with children. It is helpful to run activities by others prior to use as well. It is also helpful for children to have a sample of the activity being used. We recommend having several examples of finished activities to avoid children simply copying the sample and not getting as much from the activity as they could. Testing the activity ahead of time will help to ensure that the activity is effective and engaging for children with whom you are working.

These are just a few suggestions to consider when planning activities for groups or individual counseling. We have found in our work with children, however, that the most effective activities are developed with the specific children under your care in mind. Think about what issues the children attending your group or counseling are experiencing and consider activities that help children to make meaning, continue bonds with the deceased, problem solve, or build perspective. The remainder of this chapter provides several activities that help to experience these four modes of help.

ACTIVITIES THAT FACILITATE MEANING-MAKING

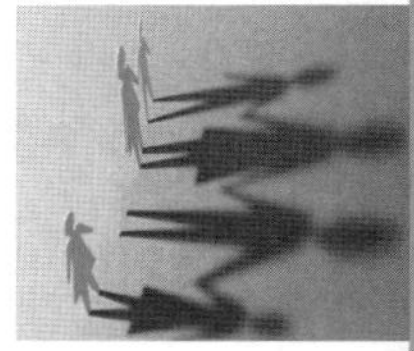

Activities, by their very nature, facilitate meaning-making because they allow the person to be creative, interact with others, or engage in ritual. More specific, though, are activities that can be used to help the child share, build, or reframe his or her narrative. On the following pages are a few samples of activities we have used over the years with children for the purpose of meaning-making. See Chapter 7 for a discussion of meaning-making.

SAMPLE ART AND WRITING ACTIVITY FOR MEANING-MAKING

Name of Activity: Writing My Story

Materials Needed: 8.5 × 11 construction paper, hole-punch, yarn or string, crayons or markers, and pen or pencil

Instructions: This activity provides children the opportunity to write about all of the circumstances surrounding the death. First, the child must identify the chapters of the story they will write. The professional can provide examples of chapters, like "My person who died," "Where I was when I was told he (or she) died," "How I felt when I found out she (or he) died," "What life was like before my person died," "What life is like now." Once you decide on the chapters, children can write the story using both words and pictures. For younger children, the professional might be the scribe (with permission from the child, of course).

Have the child select which color paper he or she wants for each of the chapters. Chapters are typically no longer than a page or two. The child might choose one color for all of the chapters or a different color for every page. This does not matter. The important thing is to allow children to be as creative as they want as they develop the narrative of the story. Have the children write the names of each of the chapters on separate pieces of paper at the top (one page per title). Let the children decide which page they would like to start with. Using techniques outlined in Chapter 8, be present with the children as they work on their storybook. This activity might take more than one session for children to complete.

Once they have completed every page of the book, stack the pages in the order they would like the chapters to be in. Then, punch holes in the left-hand margin of the stack of pages. Use the yarn or string to tie the pages together like a book. You can include a cover page if the child would like, having the child design a cover for the book. Once the book has been completed, be sure to offer the child an opportunity to read the book to you. You may also offer to read the book to the child. Let the child choose whatever he or she prefers. Offer the child the opportunity to share his or her story with parents or family (Figure 9.1).

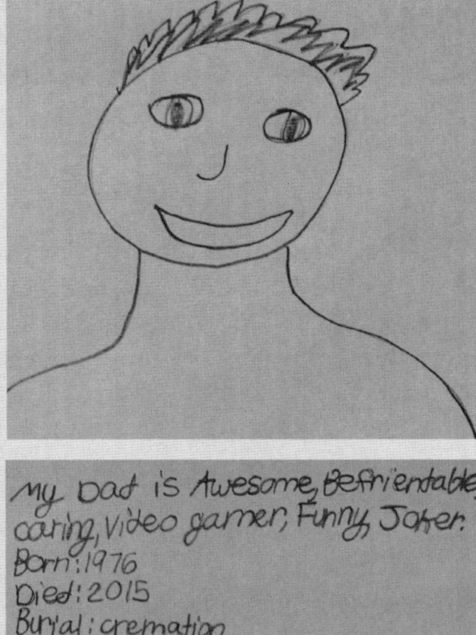

Figure 9.1 Artwork created by an older child whose dad died.

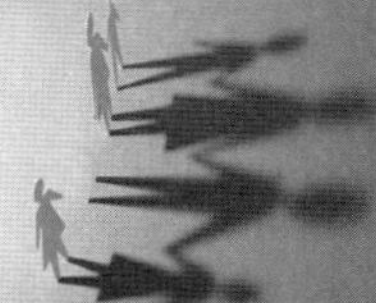

Name of Activity: Creating a World

Materials Needed and Setup: For this activity, you will need a sand tray, sand-tray sand, and sand-tray figurines (miniature people, items, objects of all sorts and types.) It is important to have a wide variety of items representing different aspects of the varied experiences that grieving children have. This could include items that represent their family, home life, leisure activities, and possessions. For example, figurines of people should represent various cultures, ages, and roles (e.g., mother, father, sibling). Figurines of people could also represent different careers, including law enforcement, doctors, emergency personnel, business people, and construction workers. It is particularly helpful to include funeral and cemetery items such as miniature coffins, urns, tombstones, and flowers. It is also important to have miniature items like alcohol bottles, cigarettes, and guns that might represent more difficult experiences. Figurines should be organized on shelves by category so they are easily accessible and available for children to peruse. If working individually with a child, place two chairs next to the sand tray so that you can be present with the child as the child creates his or her world. An alternative setup for groups can be to use small 12 × 8-inch plastic tubs. Fill each tub with sand-tray sand and place tubs on tables. Each child in the group will get a tub in which to create a world. Figurines can be displayed on shelves or tables around the edge of the room so children can easily access them.

Instructions: The professional explains to the children that the purpose of this activity is for them to create a world. Explain that they are in complete control of creating their world and everything that will inhabit their world. Before the children get up to start picking out figurines, ask the children to stop and give thought to the world they would like to create today. It could be an imaginary world. It could be the real world. It could be the world they would like to have. It could be a world that represents the past. It could be a world that represents the future. It can be any world they want it to be.

After they have a couple of minutes of reflection, instruct the children to choose the figurines and items they would like to have in their world. Explain to them that as they choose items, they might be drawn to certain items and not know why. Tell them that it is okay to have some of these items in their world. Children then select their items and bring them back to their space at the table. Once they have their items, they can begin to create a world. In an individual setting, the professional should be present with the child reflecting on the items the child has selected and is placing in the world. In a group setting, staff and volunteer facilitators should also reflect with children as they are creating a world.

Give children a 5-minute warning before ending the time for them to create the world. In an individual setting, a professional can have the child tell them about the world he or she has created. In a group setting, children can have the option to share about the world they created with others in the group. You might have everyone walk around and look at the different worlds that were created, or simply ask whether anyone would like to share about his or her world. Be mindful that sharing about the world that was created is optional for children. Some children will be eager to share, some might share even though they are hesitant, and others might not share at all. This is okay. In our experience, children who are less likely to share an art activity might be more willing to share this type of activity (Figure 9.2).

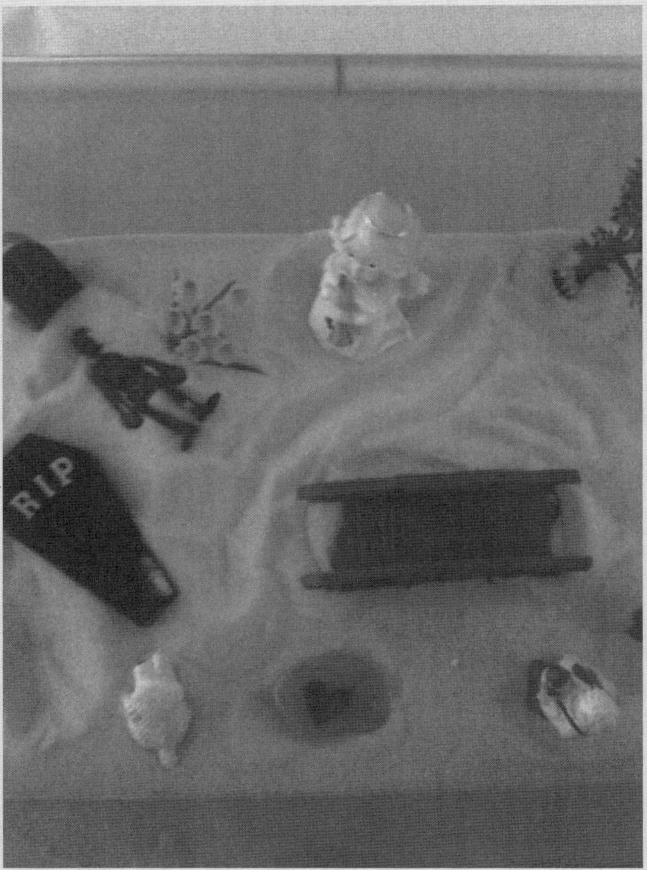

Figure 9.2 Example of a "world" created in a sand tray.

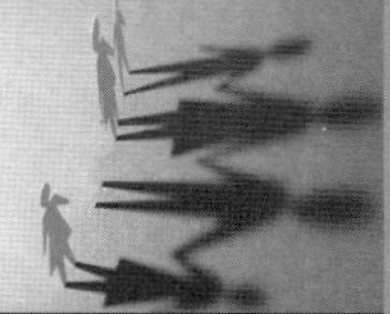

Name of Activity: Griefography

Materials Needed and Setup: To do this activity, each child will need a camera. This could be the camera on his or her parent's phone or on the child's own phone, if he or she has one. You can also use disposable cameras, if needed.

Instructions: This activity should be completed outside the group setting. It is preferable if the children have 1 or 2 weeks to take pictures from the different places where they live, go to school, and play. The professional instructs the children that they are to capture images of their world that are reflective of their grief. Images might include representations of the person who died, things that remind them of the person who died, or images that represent their grief feelings. Once they have taken the photographs, children then bring their pictures back to group to share with each other. Children are encouraged to share their photographs and the meaning they assign to those images.

An additional possibility for this activity is to give the children an option to display their photographs. This can be a major event like hosting an art show for the community, or they can be displayed on the walls of the support setting. It is important that any display of photographs is optional for children and that professionals get the proper types of permissions from children and parents. The most important thing is that children are able to construct their own narrative about the images and how these images are reflective of their unique grief experience (Figure 9.3).

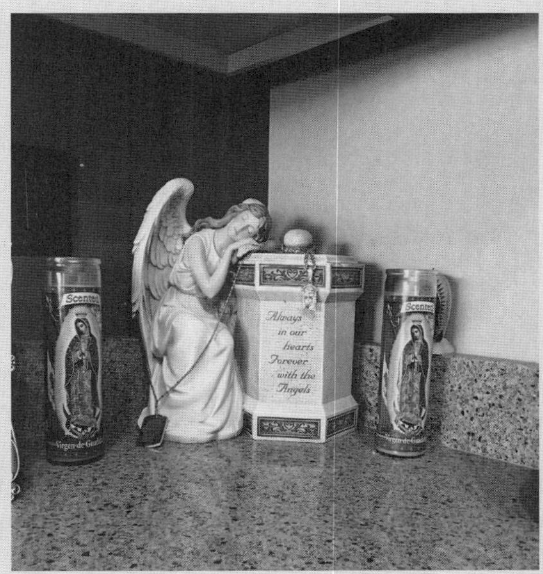

Figure 9.3 Photo taken by young child whose brother died.

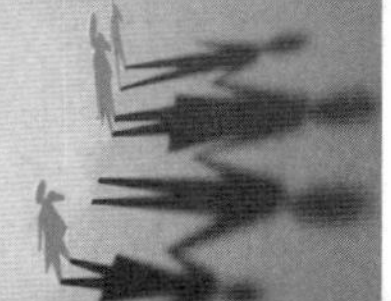

SAMPLE CANVAS-PAINTING ACTIVITY FOR MEANING-MAKING

Name of Activity: Painting My Memories

Materials Needed: Small- or medium-sized canvases; paint and paint brushes

Instructions: This activity provides children the opportunity to paint anything related to their loss. This could be the children's memories of the person who died. These memories might be good memories, but they can also be painful memories. Some children might also decide to paint about some aspect of their grief or something else that is meaningful to them. Children select a blank canvas and then decide what they would like to paint. It is optimal to have a wide array of paint colors available.

After the children have completed their paintings, they are invited to share their paintings with the rest of the group. As always, they have the option to pass if they so choose. It is helpful to allow the children to pass their paintings around if they'd like. Some children might choose to take their painting home, whereas others might want to leave theirs at the location of the support setting. The professional might choose to hang the paintings in a common area of the support setting if there is room. Children should always be given a choice about what they'd like to do with their paintings (Figure 9.4).

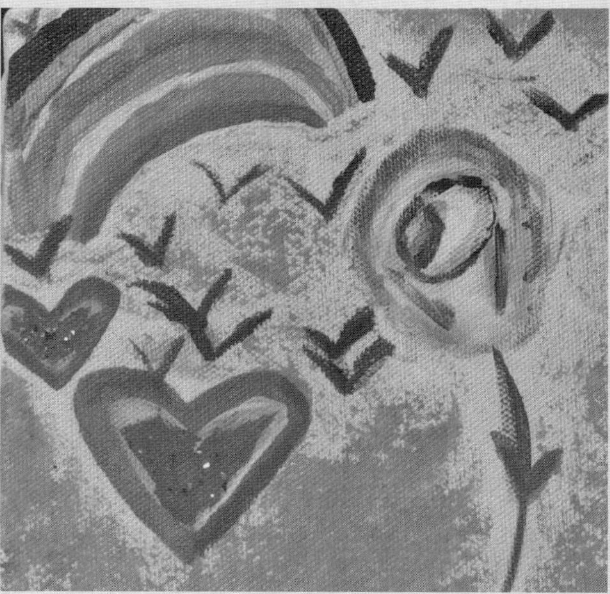

Figure 9.4 Artwork created by a teenager whose grandmother died.

ACTIVITIES THAT FACILITATE CONTINUING BONDS

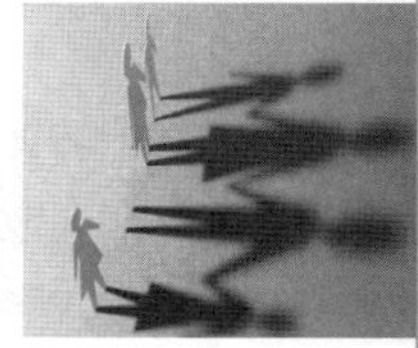

As discussed in Chapter 7, it is helpful to children to participate in activities that facilitate continuing bonds with the person who has died. These activities support a child's natural tendency to continue a connection with the person who has died, supporting a child's adaptation to the physical absence of this person in the child's life.

SAMPLE WRITING ACTIVITY FOR CONTINUING BONDS

Name of Activity: Letter to/From the Person Who Died

Materials Needed and Setup: Paper, pens, crayons, or markers; a list of sentence starters. It can sometimes be challenging for children to get sentences started. It is helpful for them to have a list of potential sentence starters or prompts on a separate sheet of paper. For example, "I want you to know…" "I really miss…" "Sometimes I am afraid…" "I am happy when…" "Some new things I'm doing are…" "I remember when…"

Instructions: This activity provides the opportunity for children to connect with the person who has died. It can be used to take care of some of the unfinished business children might have with the deceased. The professional begins by instructing children to use the sentence starters or prompts to write a letter to the deceased person. It is important that the children are able to choose their own prompts and that the content of the letter comes from them to the person who died. After they have completed their letter *to* the person who died, the children can then be instructed to complete a letter *from* the person who has died. Ask the children to think about the person and consider what this person might say to them if they could write them a letter. This allows the opportunity for children to express the encouragement or reassurance they might be missing from the deceased.

After they have completed both letters, ask the children whether anyone would like to read one of their letters (or both of them). It can be helpful for children to read or hear other children's letters read aloud. This helps children identify with others and normalizes their own feelings. Sharing their letter should be optional. Another option for this activity could be to have the child laminate the letter and take it to the cemetery or some special place where he or she feels close to the person who died. Laminating the letter can help to preserve it for the future (Figure 9.5).

SAMPLE WRITING ACTIVITY FOR CONTINUING BONDS (*continued*)

Dear, dear Momma,

I am sending this letter to you in my heart to say the one thing I probably never said enough while you were here- Thank You. Thank you for being there for me for all the practices, games and field trips. You were my biggest fan through it all and I couldn't ask for a better cheerleader. Thank you for letting me know when I was wrong and correcting me when I was being a brat. And most of all, thank you for showing me how to love.

People often tell me that I remind them of you, and to me there is no greater compliment. I admire you so much and I hope that I am living a life that would make you proud. I know you're still with me; still silently cheering me on every step of the way. I find your pennies on tails all the time, and I like to think it's you reminding me that you love me. I know I've still got some tough times ahead, but no matter what,

Forever and always your baby I'll be...

I love you.

Figure 9.5 Letter created by a teenager whose mom died.

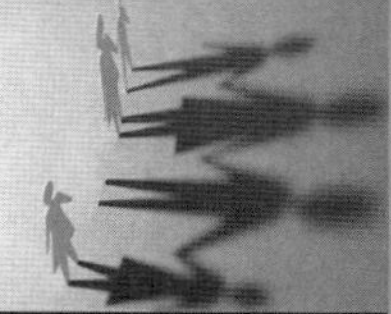

Name of Activity: Special Songs

Materials Needed and Setup: A method of playing songs in a group setting is needed. There are many options for playing music in a group setting, including using a streaming music service like Apple Music, using a child's own playlist, or accessing YouTube on the Internet.

Instructions: The week prior to this activity, professionals should let children know that they will be participating in an activity that involves music. They can explain that the children should be prepared to share a song that is meaningful to them. It could be a favorite song of the person who died or it could also be a song that reminds them of the person who died. It might be a song that helps them to feel better or even a song that helps them to feel empowered in some way.

The group leader collects the song title from each child to ensure that all of the songs are ready to be played. Before songs are played, each child is given the opportunity to introduce his or her song. The child has the option to share why he or she chose that particular song. The song is then played in full. When the song is finished, all of the children in the group are given the opportunity to share their thoughts about the song. This is repeated for each child in the group. It is helpful if the group leader introduces the activity by explaining that music is a helpful way of expressing our emotions and coping with our grief. The group leader might want to create a playlist of the group's songs that can be shared with the entire group (Figure 9.6).

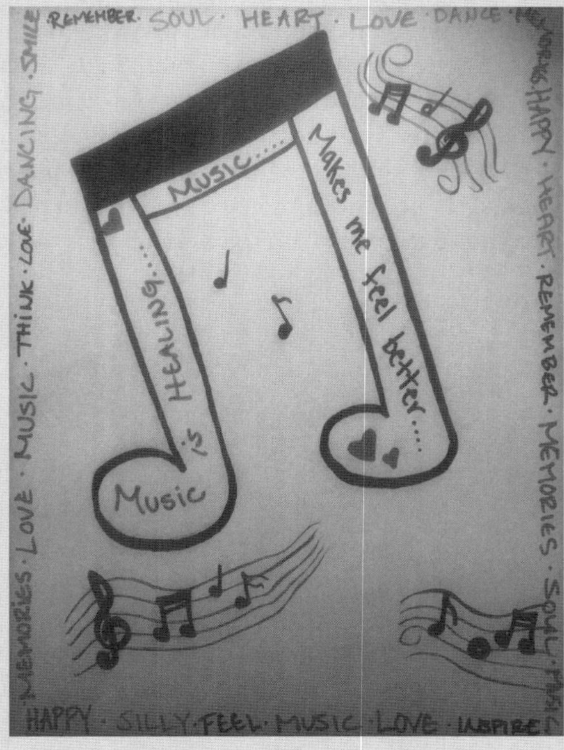

Figure 9.6 Artwork created by a teenager whose aunt died.

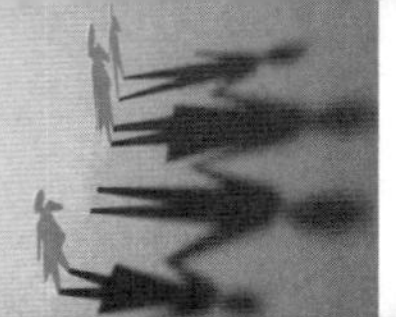

Name of Activity: Linking Objects: A Photo or Object of the Person Who Died

Materials Needed and Setup: No specific materials or setup needed

Instructions: In this activity, bereaved children bring in a photograph or object of the person who died. Some children may choose to bring in both a photograph and an object. Other children might choose to bring in just a photograph or just an object. Regardless of which items children bring, it is key that they get to decide what the item will be. Sometimes children don't have either a photograph or an object. In this case, children can draw a picture or write about the person. In a group setting, children can go around the circle and share their photograph or object with the group. They can tell anything they'd like about their items.

If they are sharing a photograph of the person who died, they can talk about the person in the photograph or any details that they know about the photograph. Sometimes children choose to bring in a photograph of their loved one alone in the photo. Other times, they might choose to bring in a photograph of themselves with the person who died. When a child brings an item in, he or she also has a choice about what he or she is going to share about that item. If the children want to, they can pass the photographs or objects around the circle. Often, children will ask each other questions about the photographs or objects. It's not uncommon for one child to remark to another, "You look a lot like your dad." Or, "Your baby sister was really cute."

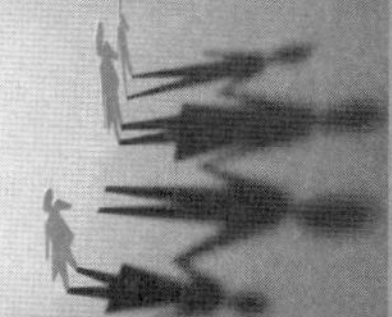

Name of Activity: Ways That I Am Similar, Ways That I Am Different

Materials Needed and Setup: Paper, pens, crayons, or markers

Instructions: This activity provides the opportunity for children to remember the person who has died while thinking about ways that they are similar to the person and ways that they are different. Growing up, children often compare themselves to other people in their family. This comparison can sometimes increase after someone dies. Once the children have chosen the paper and preferred writing instruments, the professional should ask them to think about ways that they are similar to the person who died. They can also be instructed to think about things that they have in common with that person. Next, ask the children to think about ways that they are different than the person who died. Have the children think about things like physical appearance, personality traits, behavior, ability, likes or dislikes. The group leader can give the children examples of ways that they might be similar and ways that they might be different.

Keep in mind that some children might want to write about their similarities/differences and some might prefer to draw a picture. Other children will choose to use a combination of both words and drawings. Some children might prefer to make a list with the headings "Similarities" and "Differences" at the top. After they have completed their activity, allow the children to share them with the group if they so choose. Allow children to pass their papers around the room to the other children, if they'd like to. When children hear about the similarities and differences that others have, this helps them to identify with others and normalizes their own feelings. Sharing their activity should be optional (Figure 9.7).

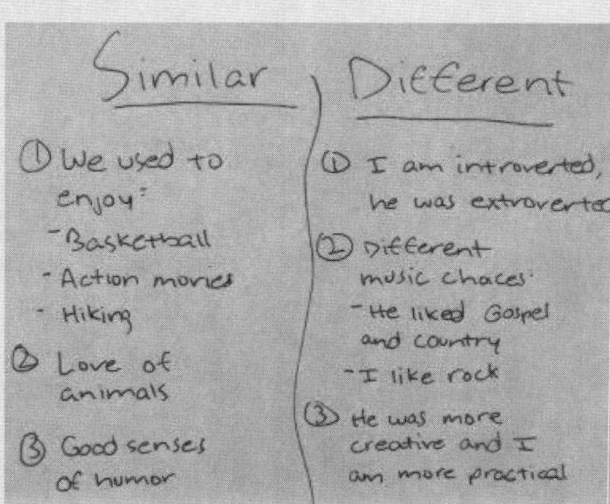

Figure 9.7 Similarities and differences list created by a teenager whose dad died.

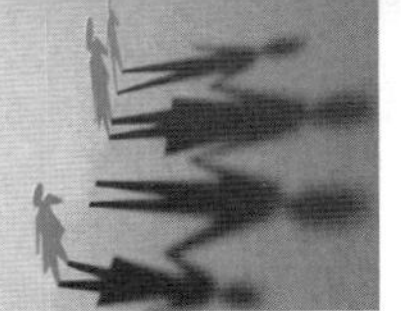

ACTIVITIES THAT FACILITATE PROBLEM SOLVING

It is important to provide opportunities for children to process some of the challenges resulting from the death of someone in their lives. As children learn to process and solve problems in their daily lives, they strengthen self-confidence and belief in their ability to navigate the many challenges that life will bring. For more about problem solving see Chapter 7.

SAMPLE WRITING ACTIVITY FOR PROBLEM SOLVING

Name of Activity: Things That People Say

Materials Needed and Setup: Paper, pens, crayons, or markers

Instructions: Have children think of some of the things that people said to them after the death that they thought were hurtful. This might even include statements that were intended to be helpful. It is important to have the children write the statements down. After the children have completed their lists, invite them to share with others in the group if they would like. Children will find this very entertaining and they often have many of the same statements listed. Once everyone has had a chance to share, the leaders should transition to the second part of the activity, which is to problem solve how to respond to someone when he or she says hurtful things. Select one of the statements and use this to set up a scenario that you can use to walk the children through the problem-solving model presented in Chapter 8. Make sure children think of a variety of options about how to respond when people say hurtful things (Figure 9.8).

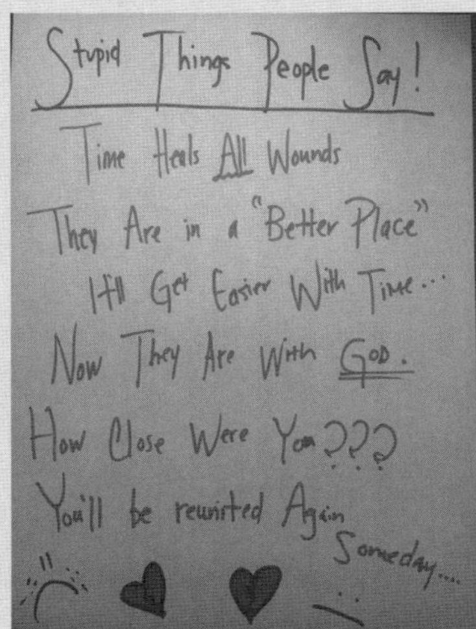

Figure 9.8 Things That People Say list created by a teenager whose friend died.

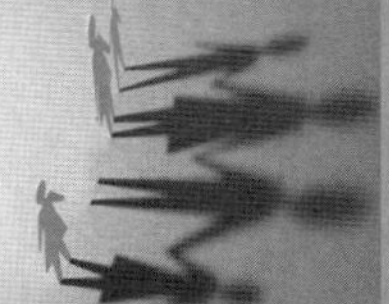

SAMPLE ART AND WRITING ACTIVITY FOR PROBLEM SOLVING

Name of Activity: Bursting With Emotions

Materials Needed and Setup: Paper, pens, crayons, or markers

Instructions: The feelings associated with grief can be quite challenging for children. It is important to normalize the feelings bereaved children might be having. The purpose of this activity is not to problem solve ways to get rid of sadness; it is to problem solve ways to cope with sadness in healthy ways. This activity accomplishes two goals, expression of feelings and ideas for coping with those feelings.

Children are instructed to draw and color a volcano. The leader might want to provide a sample picture of a volcano for the children. Children are then asked to think of feelings they have experienced since the death. They are then asked to write each of these feelings bursting out of the volcano. This is a particularly impactful image with which the children can identify. They will also notice many of the feelings they are experiencing are included in the pictures of other children. This helps to normalize what they are feeling.

Next, the leader can select some of the feelings that the children have in common. As a group, the leader can ask the children to share what types of things they do when they are feeling these feelings. They can ask the children to reflect on which reactions are helpful and which reactions are not so helpful. They can lead a discussion with the children about ideas for coping with certain feelings in ways that are healthy. It is important that the leader give children time to reflect on their ideas and suggestions. For ideas about healthy coping, see Chapter 6 (Figure 9.9).

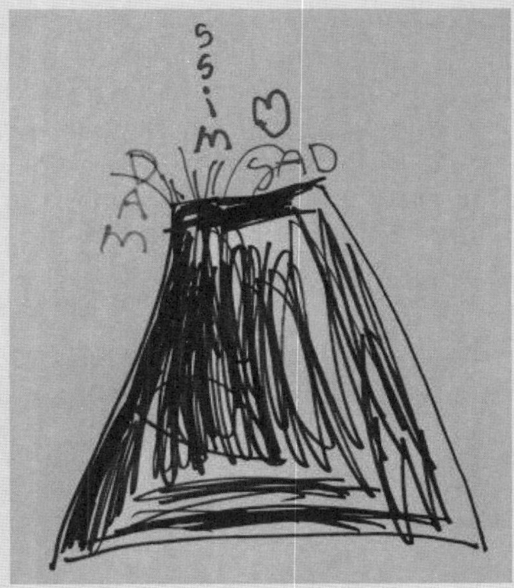

Figure 9.9 Volcano created by a younger child whose cousin died.

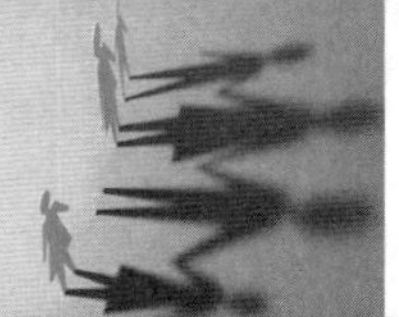

SAMPLE SHARING ACTIVITY FOR PROBLEM SOLVING

Name of Activity: Coping With Grief Triggers

Materials Needed and Setup: Sticky notes, pens, or markers

Instructions: *Grief triggers* is a widely used term to describe the experience of grief reminders that occur all around grieving people. Grief triggers typically remind the griever of the person who died or other painful aspects of the grief experience. Grief triggers can happen at any time or in any place. Often, a child's grief is triggered when he or she least expects it or when he or she is unprepared to deal with the grief that the trigger produces. Grief triggers are sensory based. Some examples of grief triggers could be a song on the radio, the smell of the air during a particular time of year, people who look like or remind the child of the deceased, or driving by particular locations associated with the person who died. This activity provides children with the opportunity to identify their own grief triggers and problem solve ways to cope with them.

The leader distributes 10 to 12 sticky notes to each child in the group. Children are instructed to think about things that have triggered their grief. The leader might give the children examples to help them to begin thinking about their own grief triggers. Children are asked to write these triggers on the notes, writing one trigger per note. Once all of the children are done, they are then asked to stick the notes on a designated wall in the room without covering up anyone else's. It is important to make sure that each sticky note is clearly displayed. The leader, along with help from the children, begins grouping the sticky notes, such as songs on the radio, smells in the air, the seasons, people who remind them of their person and special occasions, to name a few. These groupings then provide a context for a problem-solving discussion with the children. The leader can then use the problem-solving model from Chapter 8 to take the children through a discussion of ways that they can cope with grief triggers as they occur (Figure 9.10).

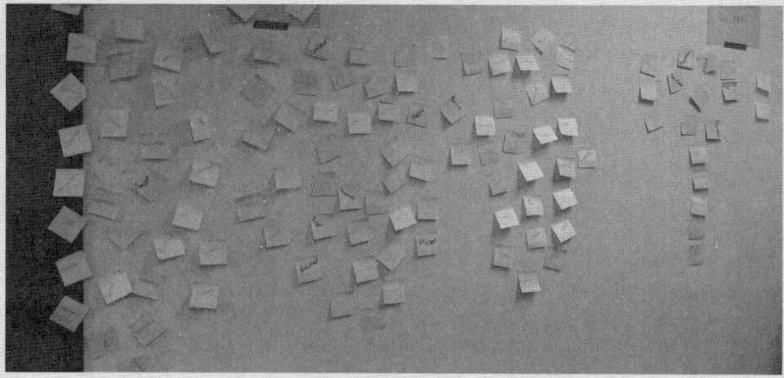

Figure 9.10 Coping With Grief Triggers activity created by a group of teenagers.

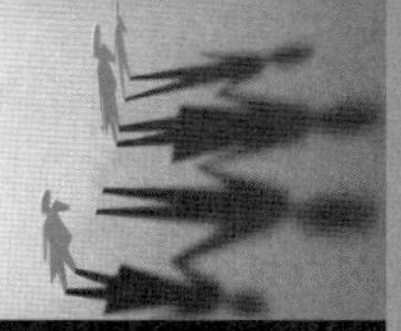

Name of Activity: Big Fears, Little Fears

Materials Needed and Setup: Paper of all sizes—some large sheets and some smaller sheets; pens, crayons, or markers

Instructions: Have children think about and discuss fears that they have. Explain to the children that most people have big and little fears. Some big fears can cause children a lot of worry, but smaller fears can also cause concern. Professionals should ask children to think about the fears or worries that they have. Next, ask the children to think about which fears are big fears and which fears are little fears. Then the professional should invite them to write their big fears on the larger piece (or pieces) of paper and to write their little fears on the smaller pieces of paper. It is up to the children to choose which fears they consider big and which fears they consider little.

After the children have completed their activity, invite them to share with others in the group if they so choose. Hearing the fears of other children helps to normalize their own fear. One of the common fears that bereaved children have is that someone else in their life might die or that they might die. Another common fear is a fear of illness or a fear of being in the dark. Professionals should discuss the fears that the group has in common and also the fears that are different. Building connections with fears that children share can be very helpful, especially when children realize that they are not the only ones who are worried about someone else dying. Discuss ways that the children can cope with their fears as they arise (Figure 9.11).

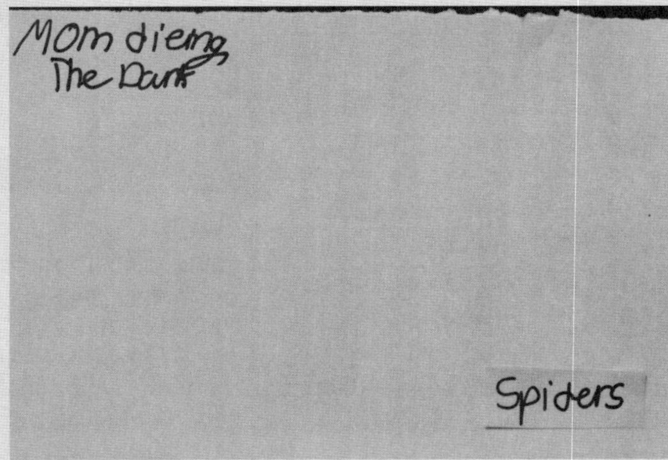

Figure 9.11 Fears listed by a younger child whose dad died.

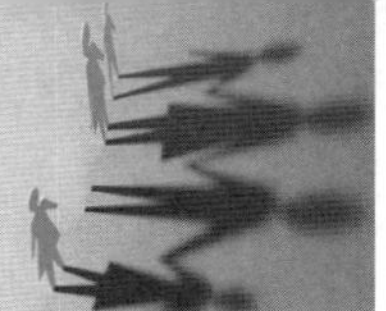

ACTIVITIES THAT FACILITATE PERSPECTIVE BUILDING

The death of someone in a child's life challenges his or her perception of how the world works. It is common for children to build their own perspective about what the death means to their lives. Providing children with opportunities to participate in activities that facilitate perspective building can broaden their understanding of their situation and offer alternative ways to view it. For more on perspective building, see Chapter 7.

SAMPLE ART AND WRITING ACTIVITY FOR PERSPECTIVE BUILDING

Name of Activity: Walking in My Grief-Filled Shoes

Materials Needed and Setup: Colored paper, pens, crayons, markers, and scissors

Instructions: Perspective-building activities are important to help children step back from the situations they are in and to gain additional insight into their family and surrounding circumstances. It also provides an opportunity to look at situations from different angles or points of view. The leader invites the children to take a piece of paper and trace the outline of a shoe. After they have traced the shoe, they use the outline to cut out a paper shoe. Once this is done, the children can draw or write anything on the cutout of the shoe that describes what it's like to be them for a day. How would someone feel if they were walking in the child's grief-filled shoes? Children are invited to go into as much or as little detail as they would like.

After the children have completed the activity, they are invited to share their shoes with the rest of the group. As always, they have the option to pass if they choose to. It is helpful to allow the children to pass their shoes around if they'd like. Once the shoes are completed, the professional might

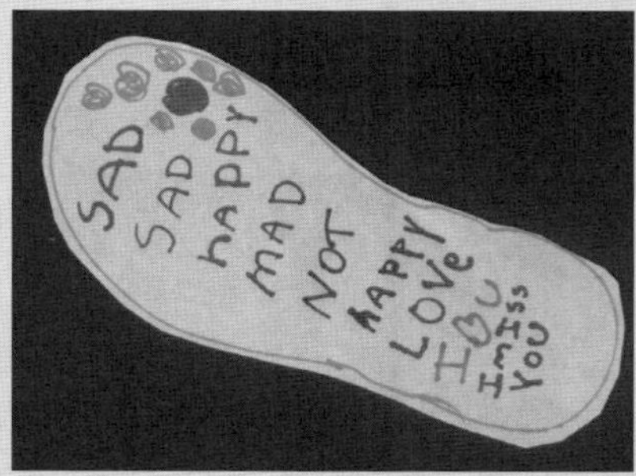

Figure 9.12 Shoe created by a younger child whose grandmother died.

choose to create a path on the wall and display the shoes on this path. This is a powerful visual of both the individuality of grief and the commonality of grief. The group leader can then lead a discussion with the children about our similarities and our differences. Through this, children can gain insight into their own situation and are challenged to consider other ways to look at grief (Figure 9.12).

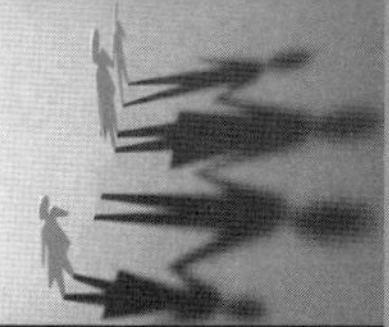

SAMPLE ART AND WRITING ACTIVITY FOR PERSPECTIVE BUILDING

Name of Activity: The People in My World

Materials Needed and Setup: Colored paper, pens, crayons, markers and scissors

Instructions: This activity offers children the opportunity to reflect on the people in their lives who are helpful and supportive. The first step is to have children trace one of their hands on paper. The leader might suggest that the children help each other trace their hands. Once they have done this, the leader asks the group to think about the people in their lives who are helpful and supportive. The leader can challenge the children to think of at least five people. Some children might have difficulty identifying people. Some might even say they do not have any people like that in their lives. This is an opportunity for the leader to help the child explore the adults in their lives that they might not be identifying.

Once the children have had a moment to consider who the helpful and supportive people in their lives are, the leader should ask them to list the name of a person who is helpful or supportive on each of the fingers of their traced hand. The children are then instructed to cut

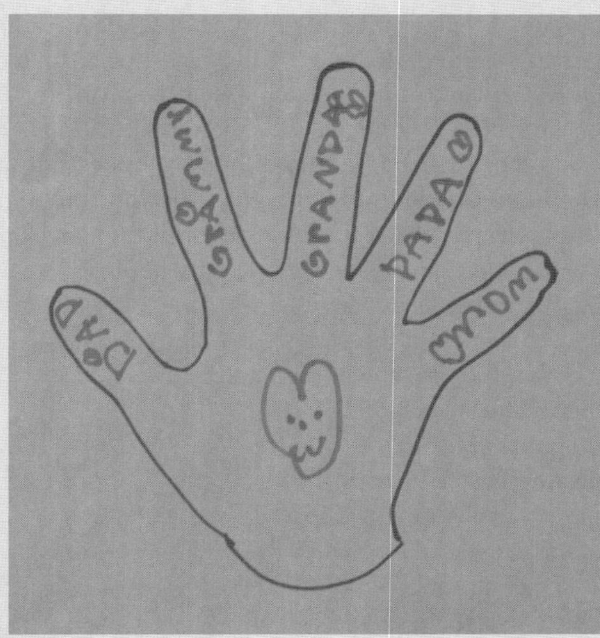

Figure 9.13 Hand created by a younger child whose cousin died.

out the outline of their hand. They are then given the opportunity to display their hand along with others on an open wall in the room. Children are invited to share about their hand and the people they have identified one at a time. Through this activity children are able to not only share about the supportive people in their lives but they can also identify the people who are helpful to others, potentially gaining insight into their own situation (Figure 9.13).

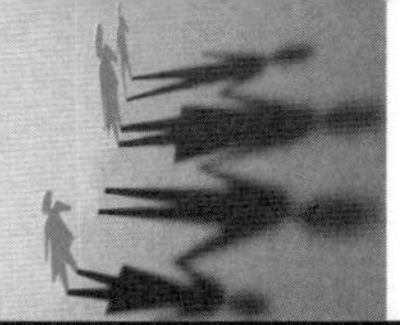

Name of Activity: Family Portrait

Materials Needed and Setup: Colored paper, pens, crayons, and markers

Instructions: Children often struggle to adapt to the changes that the death of a family member brings to their family structure. This activity provides a context for children to build perspective related to current family structures, interactions, and adjustment since the death. This activity also helps to reinforce to children that even though their family has changed, they still have a family, and families come in all shapes and sizes.

Children will select the colored paper of their choosing and whether they want to use crayons, markers, or pens. The leader asks the children to draw a picture of their family doing something together. They can give examples like playing at the park, going to the beach, or just hanging out around the house. Once the children have completed their pictures, you can ask whether any of the children would like to share their picture with the group. As children hear other children share about their families, they often talk about how things are different without the deceased person. Children will relate to others with similar family structures. After the children have had the opportunity to share, the group leader can end the activity here, or take the activity one step further.

The group leader can then ask the children to add both thoughts and words to each person in the picture. The simplest way to do this is to ask the children whether they have ever seen a thought bubble in a comic book. The leader can then draw an example of a thought bubble for the children to see. They can do the same with a speaking bubble, showing them what a speaking bubble looks like. The leaders should be prepared to have a sample portrait with thoughts and words associated with each person in the picture. This added piece allows the people in the picture to come alive and can provide additional insight into family dynamics and interactions (Figure 9.14).

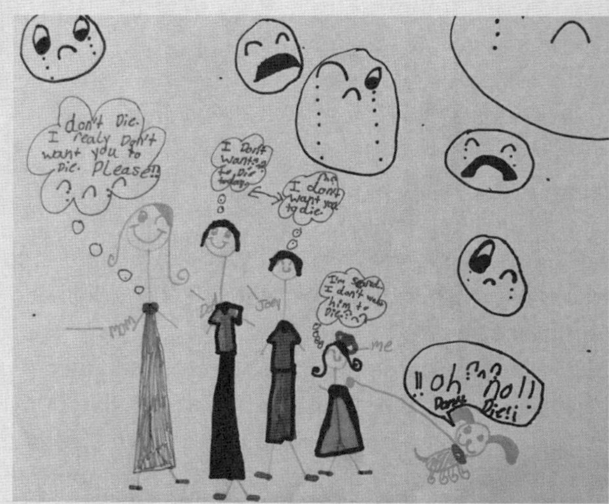

Figure 9.14 Family portrait created by a preteen whose dad died.

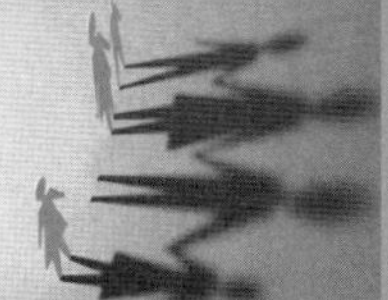

Name of Activity: What Grief Has Taught Me

Materials Needed and Setup: Paper, pens, crayons, and markers

Instructions: This activity offers children the opportunity to reflect on what they have learned as they have worked through their grief. It also offers them the chance to gain insight and perspective into the experiences of others. First, have the children think about what they have been through as a result of the death. Have them think about any new things that they have learned or observed. Give the group some examples. This is an opportunity for the professional to help the children explore their grief experiences and what they have discovered or learned from them.

Next, the children can write about what they have learned. Some children will choose to make a list, whereas others might want to put theirs in paragraph form. After they have completed the activity, invite the children to share what they have learned. Some will want to share, whereas others will not. It is optional to share and entirely up to the child. As with other activities, this activity allows children the opportunity to see what they have in common with others (or not). It also helps to normalize their grief experience and potentially gain insight into it by examining lessons learned along the way (Figure 9.15).

Figure 9.15 List of what grief has taught a teenager whose dad and brother died.

SUMMARY

The activities provided in this chapter are samples of the types of activities that professionals can employ in their work with bereaved children. Activities provide a context for children to express their unique perspectives and work through key aspects of their grief. Activities can be used for the purpose of meaning-making, continuing bonds, problem solving, and perspective building. Activities can also provide structure to the support setting. This is an important part of making sure the space is safe and child friendly. Professionals should allot time for activity planning and creativity in preparation for their group and individual sessions with children.

CHAPTER 10

Professional Accountability and Ethical Considerations

Ethics is nothing else than reverence for life.

—*Albert Schweitzer*, The Philosophy of Civilization

Childhood bereavement support is provided by a variety of professionals, including chaplains, social workers, mental health counselors, psychologists, child life specialists, nurses, school counselors, thanatologists, and educators, among others. Although many of these professions have their own licensing requirements, standards of practice, and ethical codes, there is no credentialing board for the field of childhood bereavement support. Further, there are no required courses on the subject of childhood bereavement in the fields of study for any of these professions. This often results in professionals providing bereavement support services to children and families with little to no training specific to grief and loss, leaving individuals who want to specialize in this type of work to seek out their own professional education.

Holding a professional human service degree alone, such as those listed previously, does not provide the expertise or training necessary to provide bereavement support services to children and their families. Individuals wanting to provide these types of services should seek out training above and beyond the required education for their degree or license. Individuals without the proper training or experience providing bereavement services to children and families presenting, writing, or offering advice on the subject has led to a variety of misconceptions about childhood grief. Families facing the difficult experience of losing a family member or friend benefit from seasoned, accurate information and support.

What is clear is that the knowledge and experience needed to provide bereavement support to children and their families does not rest with one particular profession. Nor does the formal training for any one particular profession offer comprehensive training in the area of childhood bereavement support. Therefore, it is important for us to discuss the issue of professional accountability and ethical considerations when working with bereaved children and their families in order to offer a framework for standards for this important and needed type of support. Keep in mind that first and foremost professionals should adhere to the standards and ethical considerations as laid out by the governing body of their profession. The following are suggested standards and ethical considerations based on our years of experience working with bereaved children and their families. Although specific credentialing or a governing board does not exist, there are standards that should be considered in order to give bereaved children and families the best care possible.

STANDARDS OF PRACTICE

Organizations that provide support to bereaved children should establish written, agreed-upon standards of practice to which program staff and volunteers are held accountable. These standards should provide a clear description of services and guidelines regarding interactions between participants and support providers both inside and outside of the support setting. Over the past 50 years, individuals working with bereaved people have formed associations and gathered to share insight from both research and practice. Because of this there is an extensive body of literature on the subject of death, dying, and bereavement to which professionals can turn to learn the most current information regarding bereavement support practices.

Education and Training

Established in 1976, The Association for Death Education and Counseling (ADEC) has provided a professional home to individuals providing support to the bereaved. ADEC offers a Code of Ethics that professionals should bear in mind when they are considering an ethical course of action (Meagher & Balk, 2013). In addition, ADEC offers certification in thanatology through their Certified in Thanatology (CT) and Fellow in Thanatology (FT) programs. These certifications require that a professional provide a specific number of hours of experience in and attend a specified level of training particular to the bereavement, death, and dying field. Educational offerings are provided through their online education program and in person at their annual conference on death, dying, and bereavement.

Professionals providing support to bereaved children began gathering in 1996 for the Symposium on Childhood Grief, which has provided education and training specific to childhood bereavement support for the past 20 years. The National Alliance for Grieving Children (NAGC) grew out of the Symposium on Childhood Grief and was established in 2004. The NAGC has developed suggested standards of practice for the field of childhood bereavement support, which were developed and agreed upon by leaders from across the childhood bereavement field. These leaders represent the variety of professions mentioned previously. In addition, the NAGC provides educational opportunities through their online education programs, as well as the annual Symposium on Childhood Grief.

The Dougy Center for Grieving Children offers a summer institute where professionals can receive education and training on how to run a support group for grieving children and families. Their training is an intensive weeklong experience where participants are given all of the information about setting up and facilitating a support program in their local area. Over the past 30 years, hundreds of individuals have attended this training and hundreds of bereavement support programs have been established across North America as a result of their efforts.

Also, the National Hospice and Palliative Care Organization (NHPCO) and the Hospice Foundation of America (HFA) both provide a variety of educational opportunities (online and in person) throughout the year. Though many of their offerings are specific to hospice care, both organizations offer topics specific to childhood grief support. Through organizations like these, as well as standards of practice and training through ADEC and the NAGC, professionals have a variety of options when considering standards for practice and for seeking education and training specific to childhood bereavement.

Staff Education Recommendations

As discussed in Chapter 8, children's bereavement support might take place in a number of professional settings. Further, those providing care might come from a variety of human service professions. Whatever the background of the care provider, we recommend that staff working directly with bereaved children and families hold at least a master's degree or higher in human service education (e.g., psychology, counseling, social work, child life). In cases in which a person has a bachelor's degree or is an intern student, we recommend that this individual be under the supervision of a master's-level practitioner. Holding a master's degree, however, is only a minimal recommendation in our opinion.

Understanding childhood grief and how to help children who are bereaved is not required learning for any master's-level human service degree. Therefore, we recommend that professionals providing direct support seek continuing education specific to understanding and supporting bereaved children and their families. As previously mentioned, ADEC, NAGC, NHPCO, and HFA all provide educational sessions online and through conferences specific to bereavement and end of life. This also includes sessions specific to childhood grief. In addition to these programs, certifications and degrees in thanatology are available through a number of institutions, including ADEC, Marian University, and Arizona State University, to name a few. A complete listing can be found on the NAGC website at childrengrieve.org.

Professional Development

Professional development is an ongoing process. Each year offers new research, new ideas, and new, innovative approaches to supporting bereaved people. Depending on the size and scope of an organization or program, providing opportunities for professional development of staff might be difficult. However, professional development should be a priority for those offering support and counseling to bereaved children and their families. In many ways formal bereavement support and counseling is a growing and changing field. New research is being conducted and practice-based evidence to provide effective support and counseling models for supporting bereaved children is determined. Continuing education can provide fresh perspectives, offer further support to existing ideas, and reignite personal passion for supporting people during difficult times.

Volunteer Screening, Training, and Support

Organizations using volunteers have an obligation to train their volunteers in key aspects of understanding childhood bereavement and how to provide support to grieving children. It is not enough to solely provide an orientation training to volunteers; it is also important to offer continued training for both new and existing volunteers. New information and research continue to inform our understanding of how grief impacts the lives of children and how we can help them. Keeping both your staff and volunteers up to date regarding this information is important to the services provided to those under your care.

It is also important to properly screen volunteers. This begins with screening volunteers working directly with bereaved children using mandatory background checks. This, however, is only one aspect of screening volunteers. Providing direct support to bereaved children and their families can be physically, emotionally, and mentally draining at times. Physically, volunteers have to be prepared to follow children in their play. Children have a lot of energy and this can be taxing on individuals with less physical stamina. There are also many emotionally charged stories and expressions that can trigger thoughts and emotions in those providing direct care. This can be particularly true for individuals who are dealing with their own grief over the death of someone in their lives. Screening for readiness to provide support should be part of volunteer orientation. This will allow volunteers to explore their own grief and their readiness to be with children in a support setting.

Informed Consent and Description of Services

The parent or legal guardian of children attending individual support, peer support groups, or grief camps should be provided a clear description of services being offered. Although this description should include your mission statement, it should also detail the organization's values, the process used to provide bereavement support, and the credentials or experience of those providing the care. This should also offer a clear description of services, including when services end. We should be prepared to provide appropriate referrals when the needs of a particular child might be outside our scope of services. What we say we are providing bereaved children and families in the way of support is the contract we make with those children and families under our care. Families should be aware of what they are signing their children and themselves up for when agreeing to attend bereavement support with you or your organization.

Mission, Vision, Values

Having a clear mission and vision for your organization or program, as well as established values will help to guide your programs and practices. Volunteers, staff, and even those attending support should all understand why your organization exists and what your organizations stands for as a shared group. Services provided should fit within the mission and vision of your organization. Services should also reflect the values of your organization. For example, in our practice we place a value on the worth and autonomy of every child. This means we believe that each child has the ability to experience and cope with his or her grief in whatever way feels most natural to that child. This value guided many of our approaches to supporting bereaved children, specifically our practice to provide children with a variety of options in the counseling and support setting. If you do not already have a mission, vision, or value statement, consider how services are delivered to children and build these statements out of your existing practice. Mission, vision, and value statements can serve as the shared contract you have with one another as caregivers and with the children and families under your care.

Program Delivery

Person Centered

Because grief is a personal, transitional experience for children, support and counseling should be client centered. Carl Rogers's person-centered approach to therapy has served as a model for understanding that the supporter and the person seeking support are equal partners. Further, Rogers argued that people seeking support possess their own solutions and that the counseling or support environment provides the setting for them to discover these solutions for themselves. We have found that a person-centered approach to supporting bereaved children and their families is most effective for establishing rapport and creating a setting that is conducive to self-exploration and self-realization. Even programs that might be more directive or curriculum based should provide options and allow those attending support to express openly and to seek solutions that feel most natural to them.

Privacy

An important part of building trust in the support relationship is respecting the privacy of those attending supportive interventions. This is accomplished in a variety of ways. First, we recommend establishing the expectation that participants are allowed to share as little or as much as they want. Many programs establish a rule that if someone doesn't want to share, they do not have to share. We have had children attend counseling and groups who did not talk for months. The reality is that there are more ways that children are supported than simply talking about their grief. This also protects a child's right to his or her own privacy and to share whatever, if anything, the child feels comfortable sharing.

Another way to protect the privacy of those attending support is to have a confidentiality policy with volunteers and staff. Stories shared in a group or counseling setting by participants should be held in confidence by the staff and volunteers working with those children and families. This also means not sharing things children talk about in the support setting with parents or caregivers. The only exception to this is if children share information or plans that could cause harm to themselves or others. Then confidentiality *must* be broken and parents notified. Otherwise, there should be an understanding that what it said in the support setting stays in the support setting.

A third way we can protect the privacy of those attending support is to have a confidentiality guideline we promote with group members. Although we cannot guarantee that all members of the group will keep information shared in the group confidential, it is still important to set the expectation. As previously mentioned, trust is an important component to creating a safe space for children to express their grief.

Environment

As discussed in detail in Chapter 8, an important standard for program delivery is ensuring that the environment is child friendly, with activities and options appealing to children. Equally important is that the environment has a variety of options for children. Though offering variety can be challenging in some settings, it should still be a standard of program delivery. This will allow children to express their grief in the way that feels most natural to them. Also, providing an environment that is warm and free from pressure or coercion allows children the opportunity to share and interact with others on their own terms.

ACCOUNTABILITY

Whether we are providing individual support, group support, or camps for bereaved children and their families, it is important that those delivering services are accountable to someone outside of themselves.

Staff Supervision and Care

Staff and volunteers providing support services to children and families should be supervised by a master's-level human services professional on staff with experience in the field of childhood bereavement support and knowledge regarding appropriate referrals for issues outside the scope of the organization. In the case of smaller volunteer-run organizations or those with limited staff, the board of directors should retain the services of a master's-level human service professional consultant to provide supervision and referral.

Those providing individual and family support who are not connected with a particular organization should be accountable to their own profession's licensing board. In the case of professionals working in an organization without a licensing board, we suggest establishing a supervisory relationship with another professional from your field, or a master's-level human service professional for the purpose of supervision, accountability, and referral.

Volunteer Supervision and Care

Death, dying, and bereavement are shared human experiences. To work in compassionate support services requires individuals who are able of empathizing with the stories and situations of those seeking support. Because of this, it is normal for professionals providing bereavement support to children and their families to identify with and form bonds with those under their care.

Although these types of connections are important to be able to provide support and understanding to the individuals under care, it is also important that professional boundaries are in place to avoid dual relationships and conflicts of interest.

Dual relationships and conflicts of interest can be defined as any relationship in which multiple roles might compromise the integrity of the professional providing support and the individual seeking support. This might include business relationships, romantic relationships, or friendships that contaminate the professional relationship. Clear guidelines should be set within organizations and programs to protect the bereavement support environment. Staff and volunteers should avoid pursuing relationships with those attending support services outside the support setting. This will protect the interests of the children and families receiving services, as well as the service providers.

Referral

Knowing where your services begin and where they end is equally important. Organizations or individuals providing bereavement support services to grieving children and families should be able to provide appropriate referrals when children are exhibiting symptoms outside the scope of grief. It is important to provide families with information about where to get the right kind of help for the struggles parents or children might be experiencing. Being a part of a local mental health network, or social service coalition, is a great way for bereavement support professionals to be part of the greater support community. The relationships forged through participating in regular meetings with other professionals create a community of support where collaboration and a variety of expertise are made available to families.

Language and Labeling

The language we use to talk about grief can have a direct impact on the way children perceive their situation. Children and their families often seek support because they are struggling with many confusing thoughts and feelings. Parents are worried that what their children are experiencing might be detrimental or damaging. In turn, children might worry about their parents and the changes at home since the death. Bereavement support professionals have a unique opportunity to provide insight into how grief manifests itself in the lives of children and coping strategies for dealing with the associated thoughts and feelings.

Because of this, professionals should use clear, easy-to-understand language when educating families about grief. Heavily clinical terms can be confusing for families and can also paint a picture of grief as being a pathology that must be treated. As mentioned in Chapter 1, there is an ongoing debate among mental health professionals regarding the diagnosis of certain manifestations of grief. This debate has led some to create lists of certain grief-related symptoms that, in their opinion, denote a special type of grief experience requiring specialized treatment.

Currently, the *Diagnostic and Statistical Manual of Mental Disorders,* Fifth Edition (*DSM-5*; American Psychiatric Association, 2013) has included one such construct in their "for further study" section: persistent complex bereavement disorder (PCBD). This disorder was derived from several different schools of thought, including complicated grief and prolonged grief proponents. There are different philosophical opinions surrounding this issue. Diagnosing certain types of bereavement experiences as in need of "special" treatment, can provide a context for downplaying other types of bereavement experiences as "normal," leading the helping community to falsely believe that children not exhibiting the special symptoms needed for diagnosis are "okay" and not in need of support.

We would do well to remember that the field of childhood bereavement support came about, in part, as a reaction to the mischaracterization that children do not grieve and will be fine if left alone and allowed to move on. This created an environment in our society around death in which children were excluded from end-of-life rituals and left to grieve alone. They were touted as resilient and able to "bounce back." As a field, we should consider the ethical implications of creating a special diagnosis for certain types of grief reactions, as well as the long-term impact this will have on providing children and their families a safe place where they can be supported while adapting to a very difficult reality in their lives. It has been our experience that the signs and symptoms assigned to constructs like complicated grief, prolonged grief, or PCBD are rather common experiences among bereaved children and adults. This, in our opinion, serves to further confuse bereaved people and primarily benefits the practitioner providing the specified form of treatment to remedy the condition.

Misconceptions

Far too often we hear human service professionals sharing misinformation or old and outdated ideas about grief on the news or in journal articles. There is a large body of literature written about childhood bereavement today, yet many professionals continue to discuss grief in terms of stages, or talk about grieving children as "resilient" and better off if left alone to "bounce back" on their own.

Therefore, as bereavement support professionals, we have an ethical obligation to stay abreast of new developments and insights into childhood grief and how to help. Professional development is an ongoing process and we should never stop seeking education and new findings related to helping bereaved children. In turn, we should also work to correct misconceptions and provide good, accurate information to other professionals, as well as families regarding childhood grief and how to help grieving children.

SUMMARY

Dealing with the death of a person in their life is difficult for children. Grief is not a one-time experience, but a process of adapting to new realities and understandings as a child grows, develops, and matures. The care we provide bereaved children matters, from the language we use about grief to the environment we create in our support settings. It is important that we establish and follow clear standards of care and that we consider the ethical implications around how we interact with and support children and their families. Death is a universal reality we will all experience. Let us support each other with the care, professionalism, kindness, and personal human touch that we all need in the darkest moments of our lives.

REFERENCES

American Psychiatric Association. (2013). *Diagnostic and statistical manual of mental disorders* (5th ed.). Arlington, VA: American Psychiatric Publishing.

Meagher, D., & Balk, D. E. (Eds.). (2013). *Handbook of thanatology: The essential body of knowledge for the study of death, dying, and bereavement.* New York, NY: Routledge.

Index